A SELF-INSTRUCTIONAL GUIDE TO
ORAL SURGERY IN GENERAL DENTISTRY

edited by

James R. Hooley, DDS
Robert J. Whitacre, MS, DDS

CHAPTER ONE

INSTRUMENTS USED FOR ORAL SURGERY

(ISBN #0-89939-010-2)

by

James R. Hooley, DDS
Robert J. Whitacre, MS, DDS

A SELF-INSTRUCTIONAL GUIDE TO ORAL SURGERY IN GENERAL DENTISTRY

(Complete Series ISBN #0-89939-000-5)

edited by

JAMES R. HOOLEY, DDS
Chairman
Dept. of Oral & Maxillofacial Surgery
School of Dentistry
University of Washington
Seattle, Washington

ROBERT J. WHITACRE, MS, DDS
Assistant Director
Office of Instructional Development
School of Dentistry
University of Washington
Seattle, Washington

Chapter One — **Instruments Used for Oral Surgery**
(ISBN #0-89939-010-2)

Two — **The Removal of Teeth**
(ISBN #0-89939-020-X)

Three — **Medications Used in Oral Surgery**
(ISBN #0-89939-030-7)

Four — **Surgical Complications**
(ISBN #0-89939-040-4)

Five — **Asepsis in Oral Surgery (Dental Asepsis)**
(ISBN #0-89939-050-1)

Six — **Assessment of and Surgery for Impacted Mandibular Third Molars**
(ISBN #0-89939-060-9)

Seven — **Pre-Prosthetic Surgery**
(ISBN #0-89939-070-6)

Eight — **Principles of Biopsy**
(ISBN #0-89939-080-3)

Nine — **Diagnosis and Treatment of Odontogenic Infections**
(ISBN #0-89939-090-0)

published by

Stoma Press, Inc.

13231 42nd Avenue NE
Seattle, WA 98125
(206) 365-2665

Printed By

ATOMIC PRESS
1421 N 34th
Seattle, WA
(206) 632-0550

Typeset By

CASTEEL TYPESETTING
18316 1st NE
Seattle, WA 98155
(206) 363-9054

INSTRUMENTS USED FOR ORAL SURGERY

by

JAMES R. HOOLEY, DDS
Chairman
Dept. of Oral & Maxillofacial Surgery
School of Dentistry
University of Washington
Seattle, Washington

ROBERT J. WHITACRE, MS, DDS
Assistant Director
Office of Instructional Development
School of Dentistry
University of Washington
Seattle, Washington

Illustrations
by
D. Scott Phillips, DDS & Dick Eidal, DDS

Photography
by
James R. Clark

CONSULTANTS

JAMES H. QUINN, DDS
Department of Oral and
Maxillofacial Surgery
School of Dentistry
Louisiana State University
New Orleans, Louisiana

RICHARD A. SMITH, DDS
Division of Oral Surgery
School of Dentistry
University of California
San Francisco, California

RALPH G. MERRILL, DDS, MScD
Chairman
THOMAS W. ALBERT, DMD, MD
J. THEODORE JASTAK, DDS, PhD
OSCAR N. LUCAS, DDS, PhD
Department of Oral and
Maxillofacial Surgery
School of Dentistry
University of Oregon
Portland, Oregon

ROBERT A. MIDDLETON, DDS
Chairman
LUCIAN SZMYD, DMD, MS
Department of Oral Surgery
School of Dentistry
University of the Pacific
San Francisco, California

GORDON W. PEDERSEN, DDS, MSD
Department of Oral Surgery
School of Dentistry
Case-Western Reserve University
Cleveland, Ohio

ERNEST W. SMALL, DDS, MS
Chairman
Department of Oral and
Maxillofacial Surgery
School of Dentistry
University of North Carolina
Chapel Hill, North Carolina

MARTIN S. LEBOWITZ, DDS, MS
Chairman
JEFFREY L. LASKIN, DDS, MS
Department of Oral Surgery
College of Dentistry
University of Florida
Gainsville, Florida

MONTY REITZIK, BDS, FDSRCS, MB, ChB
Department of Oral Surgery
Faculty of Dentistry
The University of British Columbia
Vancouver, Canada

B. K. ARORA, BDS, DMD, MS (Oral Surgery), **FRCD, FICD**
Chairman
Department of Oral Surgery and
Anesthesia
College of Dentistry
University of Saskatchewan
Saskatoon, Canada

M. K. HAMILTON, DDS
Chairman
Department of Oral Surgery
School of Dentistry
University of Maryland
Baltimore, Maryland

GERALD R. OTT, DDS
Chairman
Department of Oral Surgery
College of Dentistry
University of Nebraska
Lincoln, Nebraska

DORAN E. RYAN, DDS, MS
Chairman
SIDNEY L. BRONSTEIN, DDS, MScD
Division of Oral Surgery
School of Dentistry
University of Colorado
Denver, Colorado

BERNARD C. BYRD, DDS, MS
Chairman
Department of Oral Surgery
School of Dentistry
Loma Linda University
Loma Linda, California

KIMBLE A. TRAEGER, DMD
RICHARD S. ALLEY, DDS, MSD
Department of Oral and
Maxillofacial Surgery
The University of Texas Health
Science Center at San Antonio
San Antonio, Texas

LAWRENCE SALMAN, DDS, MPA
Chairman
Department of Oral Surgery
College of Dentistry
New York University
New York, New York

RICHARD D. MALLOW, DDS, MS
RICHARD G. STAPLEFORD, DDS
Department of Oral Surgery
School of Dentistry
University of Detroit
Detroit, Michigan

PHILIP D. MARANO, DDS
Director
Department of Oral and
Maxillofacial Surgery
School of Dentistry
Oral Roberts University
Tulsa, Oklahoma

ERIC P. MILLAR, DDS, FRCD, FICD
Associate Director
Division of Oral Surgery
Faculty of Dentistry
McGill University
Montreal, Quebec

LEON D. FIELDER, DDS
Chairman
MARTIN STEINER, DDS
Department of Oral and
Maxillofacial Surgery
School of Dentistry
University of Louisville
Louisville, Kentucky

JOE HALL MORRIS, DDS
Chairman
HOWARD S. MISNER, DDS
Department of Oral and
Maxillofacial Surgery
College of Dentistry
University of Tennessee
Memphis, Tennessee

KENNETH W. HUGHES, DDS
Department of Oral and
Maxillofacial Surgery
College of Dentistry
University of Illinois
Chicago, Illinois

ALBERT F. STAPLES, DMD, PhD
Chairman
Department of Oral Surgery
College of Dentistry
University of Oklahoma
Oklahoma City, Oklahoma

LOUIS G. MERCURI, DDS, MS
Department of Oral and
Maxillofacial Surgery
School of Dentistry
Medical College of Virginia/
Virginia Commonwealth University
Richmond, Virginia

TABLE OF CONTENTS

MESSAGE TO LEARNER

When reading a standard textbook, it is often difficult for you to know exactly what the important content is. It is difficult to separate areas that are essential for you to understand from those that are nice to know. You may often have thought you knew the material but could not apply it when presented with the clinical situation. You may also have had a problem during examinations when instructors asked you questions that were **not** covered in your reading.

In writing this chapter, considerable time and effort have been invested in creating a feedback system for you to monitor your learning progress. We have included a section termed "overview and objectives" which states the essential kinds of performances or knowledge you can expect to gain from reading the contents and completing the study exercises. Generally, we have included a **"Pre-Test"** for each unit. The "Pre-Test" is intended to show you what you don't know about the content of the unit. It is difficult for you to see learning take place unless you have both a "before" and "after" demonstration. You should retake the pre-tests following completion of each unit.

The **study exercises** are designed for different levels of learning. The **first level** of study exercises are of the "fill in the blank" type. The blanks usually include "key" words or phrases taken from the content preceding the study exercise.

The **second level** of study exercises is designed as problem-solving tasks. Generally these take a small piece of a larger concept and allow you to focus your attention on mastery of the piece. Learning one piece at a time is similar to learning your multiplication tables. The small pieces are then assimilated into larger concepts which you can learn with ease.

The **third level** of questions are simulations of clinical problems that you will be faced with in treating patients. Having completed the previous study exercises, you should be able to adequately cope with these. These are the most important study exercises because they resemble the real world of dentistry. Through adequate analysis and planning, complications or surprises during surgery can be greatly reduced. These are similar to "story problems" in mathematics.

The study exercises are **extremely important** and you should take the time to **write the answers** in the blanks or spaces provided. You may be tempted to mentally answer the questions or skip them entirely to save time. You will **retain more of the information** you have read with much **less effort** if you take the time to write out the answers as you proceed. Considerable research in self-instructional design and learning has shown the importance of answering such study questions.

Even though the content in these chapters appears large, by no means did we intend to present the entire field of oral surgery. We intend these chapters to be your "starter kit," and strongly encourage you to obtain other reference books, journals, and materials to cover topics not discussed.

Although we have had considerable input from many people in writing these chapters, we by no means imply that these techniques, instruments or concepts are the "only way." Your oral surgeon or instructors may wish to deviate from the methods described in these chapters—especially with regards to specific clinical situations.

OVERVIEW AND OBJECTIVES

Instruments Used for Oral Surgery deals with those instruments needed to carry out oral surgery procedures in a general dental environment. Every effort has been made to minimize and simplify the instrument requirements for surgical procedures to minimize expenses for the general dentist. As a starting point, this unit will aid you in determining which instrument should be used in which general situation and how they are used when correctly applied.

Unit I — Extraction Forceps

In Unit I you will learn the basic features of extraction forceps design and how these design features are utilized in selection of a specific forceps for the removal of each tooth.

Following completion of this unit you will:

1. State the three (3) basic components of extraction forceps.
2. Describe how forceps handle design varies between the American and English style forceps in terms of:
   a. Orientation of handle toward the horizon (floor)
   b. Method of grasp for both maxillary and mandibular extractions
   c. Effects on the amount of force or leverage required
3. Describe why dental clinics prefer straight-handled over curved-handled American style forceps.
4. Describe three important considerations for forceps hinge design.
5. Diagram and describe how forceps beaks are designed to adapt to single-rooted, bifurcated, and trifurcated teeth.
6. Describe the differences in beak design necessary for forceps used in the maxillary and mandibular arches.
7. Describe the anatomy of each of the following teeth that is relevant to forceps selection and name the appropriate forceps for removal of these teeth:
   a. Maxillary anterior teeth
   b. Maxillary premolar teeth
   c. Maxillary first and second molars with crowns intact
   d. Maxillary first and second molars with crowns seriously damaged by caries, extensive restorations, or trauma
   e. Erupted maxillary third molars
   f. Maxillary root tips
   g. Maxillary primary teeth
   h. Mandibular anterior and premolar teeth
   i. Mandibular molars with crowns intact
   j. Mandibular molars with crowns seriously damaged
   k. Erupted mandibular third molars
   l. Mandibular root tips
8. Given a drawing of the human dentition showing root and crown morphology, identify the appropriate forceps to be used for extraction of each tooth.
9. Given a drawing or photograph of the following extraction forceps, give the name of the instrument and its major use in oral surgery procedures.
   a. #1 or #99-C
   b. #150 & #150-A
   c. #89 & #90 (88R & L)
   d. #53R & #53L
   e. #210-S
   f. #286
   g. #150-S
   h. #151-S
   i. #151 & #151-A
   j. #23
   k. #17
   l. #222
   m. #203
   n. #74 (or #74-N or #74 extra-N)

Unit II — Elevators

The purpose of this unit is for you to learn the basic features of the commonly used dental elevators and how elevators are used to assist in the removal of teeth. You will also learn the names for specific elevators and how they are used.

Following completion of this unit you will:

1. State the three (3) basic components of dental elevators.
2. Describe the two (2) basic types of elevators.
3. Describe the three (3) basic ways elevators are used.
4. Describe how each of the following elevators is used in the removal of teeth
   a. #30 and 31 (Cryer)
   b. #41 (Crane pick)
   c. 73 and #74 (Miller)
   d. Potts elevators
   e. #34-S and #46 (large, straight shoehorn)
   f. #301, #302 and #303
   g. Apex elevators (root picks)
5. Given a drawing or photograph of the following elevators, name the elevator and state its use in surgery
   a. #30 & #31
   b. #41
   c. #73 & #74
   d. Potts
   e. #34-S & #46
   f. #301, 302, 303
   g. Apex elevators

Unit III — Miscellaneous Surgical Instruments

The purpose of this unit is for you to learn the names and uses for other instruments commonly used during oral surgery procedures.

Following completion of this unit you will:

1. State the names of the two (2) commonly used ronguers and describe their use.
2. State the name of a surgical mallet and describe its use.
3. Describe the two (2) commonly used types of chisels and when each type is used.
4. Describe the use of curettes.
5. Name the bone file frequently used and state how this instrument is used during surgery.
6. Name and describe the use of the two (2) types of periosteal elevators commonly used in oral surgery.
7. Name an example and describe the use of a scissors.
8. Describe the use of a suture-needle holder.
9. State why hemostats should not be used as suture-needle holders.
10. Describe the surgical knife and most commonly used blades in oral surgery.
11. Describe how surgical blades should be placed on and off the surgical knife handle.
12. Name and describe the use of a tissue forceps.
13. Describe the use of transfer forceps.
14. Describe the use of a mouth prop.

15. Describe the use of mosquito hemostats in oral surgery.
16. State the function of tissue retractors.
17. Describe the two commonly used tissue retractors.
18. Describe how the suction tips used for oral surgery differ from those used in restorative dentistry.
19. State the characteristics described in the ideal rotary cutting instrument.
20. Describe three (3) rotary cutting instruments frequently used by oral surgeons and surgical clinics.
21. Name and describe the high-speed handpiece that is acceptable and practical for use in general dentistry.
22. Name and describe the use for the burs most often used during oral surgery procedures.

UNIT I

EXTRACTION FORCEPS

Introduction
Forceps Design and General Application Principles
Components of a Forceps
Maxillary Forceps
- **Anteriors: #1 and #99-C**
- **Premolars: #150 & #150-A**
- **Molar teeth: #89 & 90, 88R & L, #53R & L**
- **Third molars: #210-S**
- **Root tips: #286**
- **Primary teeth: #150-S**

Mandibular Forceps
- **Anterior and Premolar teeth: #74, #74-N & #74-extra-N, #151 & 150-A, #203**
- **Molar teeth: #23, #17**
- **Third molars: #222**
- **Primary teeth: #151-S**

PRETEST

- *Answer each question by circling the correct answer.*
- *If all questions are answered correctly, proceed to Unit II, page 28.*
- *If you do not answer all questions correctly, read and study the content of this Unit.*
- *The numbers in parentheses at the end of each question refer to the specific objective number from which this question was derived (i.e., 01-01-01 = Chapter 1 - Unit 1 - Objective 1).*

Questions:

D____ 1. *The three basic components of an extraction forceps are (01-01-01):*
- *a. finger loops, blade & tip*
- *b. handle, shank, tip*
- *c. handle, hinge & blade*
- *d. handle, hinge & beak*
- *e. none of the above*

E____ 2. *Handles of the American style forceps are (01-01-02) (01-01-06):*
- *a. grasped vertically like the English or European style.*
- *b. held in your hand with palm down for maxillary extraction.*
- *c. grasped horizontally with palm down for mandibular extractions.*
- *d. designed to provide less leverage than the English or European style.*
- *e. c and d are correct.*

Which of the following forceps beak designs will best adapt to the following teeth (01-01-05):

A____ 3. *conical rooted incisors*
B____ 4. *maxillary first molar*
D____ 5. *mandibular first molar*
A____ 6. *conical maxillary third molar*

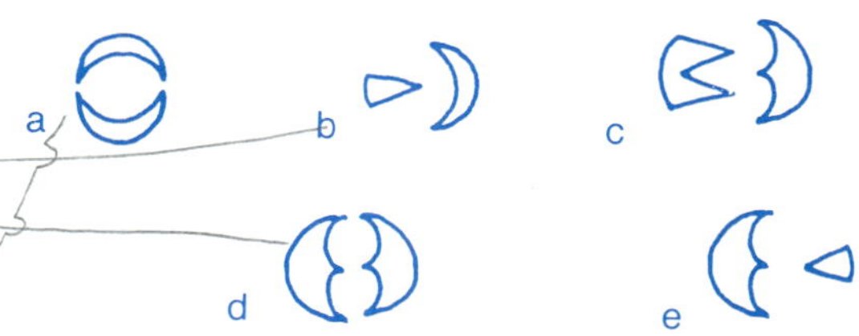

Which specific forceps is primarily designed for extraction of the following teeth (01-01-07):

E ____ 7. maxillary root tips #286
B ____ 8. maxillary central incisor #1
C ____ 9. maxillary third molars #210-S
A ____ 10. maxillary premolars #150
D ____ 11. maxillary first molar (crown intact) #53R + L

a. #150
b. #1
c. #210-S
d. #53R & L
e. ~~#222~~ 286

Which specific forceps is primarily designed for extraction of the following teeth (01-01-07):

A ____ 12. mandibular central incisor #74
E ____ 13. mandibular third molar #222
C ____ 14. mandibular first molar #23
D ____ 15. mandibular second molar with a conical root #17

a. #74
b. #151
c. #23
d. #17
e. #222

For the instruments pictured, give the number of the forceps and the purpose for which it is designed.

Name	**Designed to extract:**
1. #89-90	M. Maxillary root tips
2. #150	N. Primary maxillary teeth
3. #151	O. Mandibular first molars
4. #23	P. Mandibular conical rooted 2nd molars
5. #17	Q. Maxillary first molars
6. #150-S	R. Maxillary conical rooted 2nd molars
	S. Maxillary premolars
	T. Mandibular premolars

C ____ 16. Forceps shown in illustration (01-01-09)
a. 5 - N
b. 1 - Q
c. 4 - O
d. 3 - M
e. 6 - R

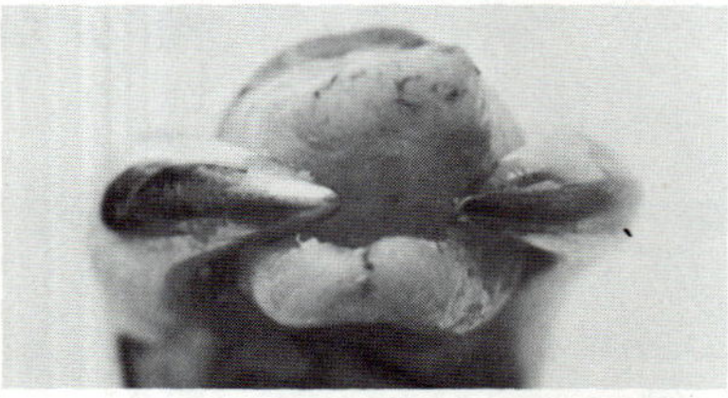

#23
MAND. 1ST MOLARS

B ____ 17. Forceps shown in illustration (01-01-09)
a. 2 - R
b. 6 - N
c. 3 - N
d. 6 - P
e. 4 - Q

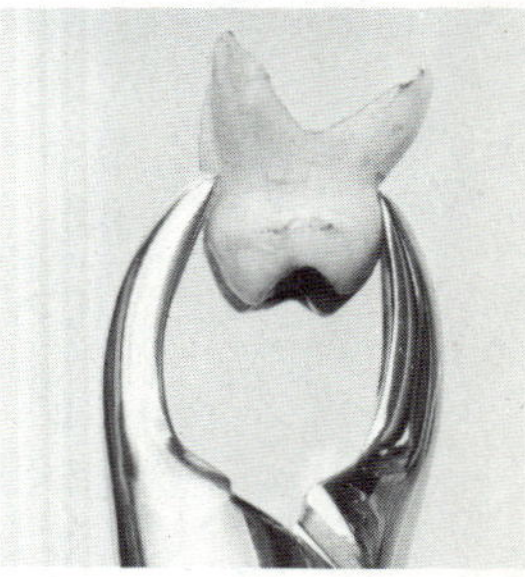

#150-S
1° MAX. TEETH

__D__ 18. *Forceps shown in illustration (01-01-09)*

a. 6 - N
b. 3 - M
c. 4 - O
d. 2 - S
e. none of the above

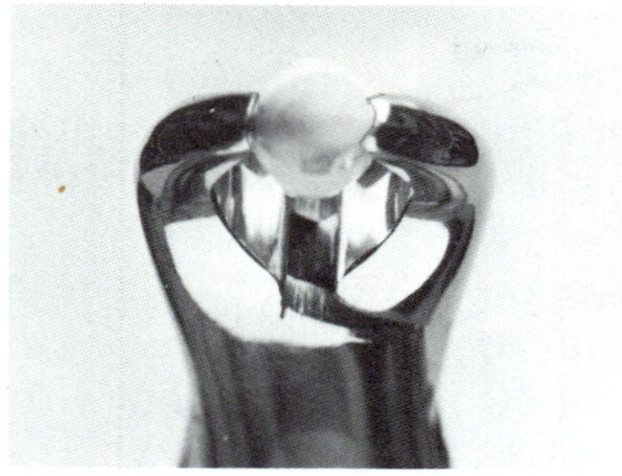

#150
MAX. PREMOLARS

__B__ 19. *Forceps shown in illustration (01-01-09)*

a. 1 - M
b. 1 - Q
c. 4 - R
d. 6 - O
e. 4 - O

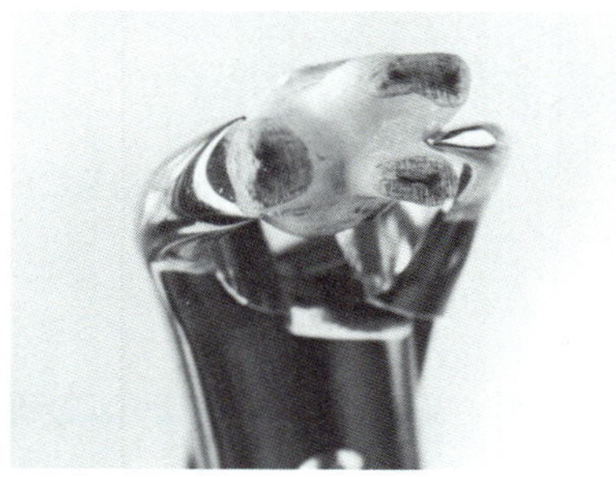

89-90
MAX. 1ST MOLARS

__B__ 20. *Forceps shown in illustration (01-01-09)*

a. 1 - T
b. 5 - P
c. 4 - R
d. 3 - R
e. 5 - Q

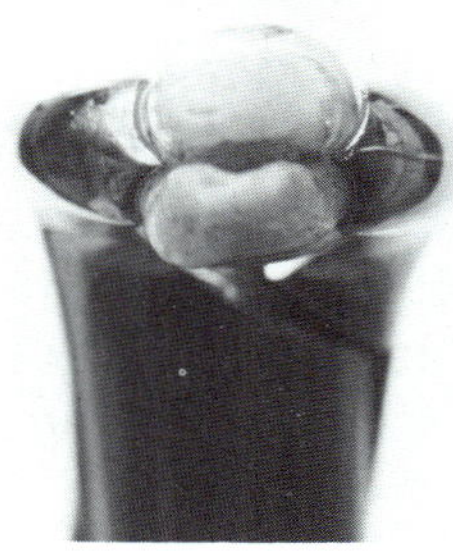

#17
MAND. CONICAL ROOTED 2ND MOLARS

Answers

1 - d	6 - a	11 - d	16 - c
2 - e	7 - e	12 - a	17 - b
3 - a	8 - b	13 - e	18 - d
4 - b	9 - c	14 - c	19 - b
5 - d	10 - a	15 - d	20 - b

INTRODUCTION TO INSTRUMENTS USED IN ORAL SURGERY

This chapter describes many of the commonly used instruments needed to perform the types of oral surgery performed by general practitioners in their offices. As a starting point for your clinical training in oral surgery you will find that a preliminary knowledge of these instruments and their basic application is helpful. As you gain additional experiences in oral surgery you, no doubt, will make substitutions or add additional instruments according to your preferences. The instruments included in this discussion have been included as a result of discussions with oral surgery faculty from several dental schools; however, complete consensus with regard to which specific instruments to include in this chapter was not possible. Thus, you may be exposed to alternatives to these specific instruments during your oral surgery training.

UNIT I

EXTRACTION FORCEPS

INTRODUCTION

The most distinctive instruments used for the removal of teeth are **extraction forceps.** The purpose of this unit is for you to learn the basic principles of instrument design as they relate to clinical use.

FORCEPS DESIGN AND GENERAL APPLICATION PRINCIPLES

Extraction forceps are forceps specially designed for removing teeth from alveolar bone. They are manufactured in a variety of configurations and styles related to both function and personal preference. We will discuss the components and design of forceps to provide you with an understanding of how instrument design affects instrument function and versatility. We will present basic principles of extraction using forceps. Then we will discuss forceps selection for extraction of specific teeth.

COMPONENTS OF A FORCEPS

The basic components of a forceps are:

- handle
- hinge
- beaks

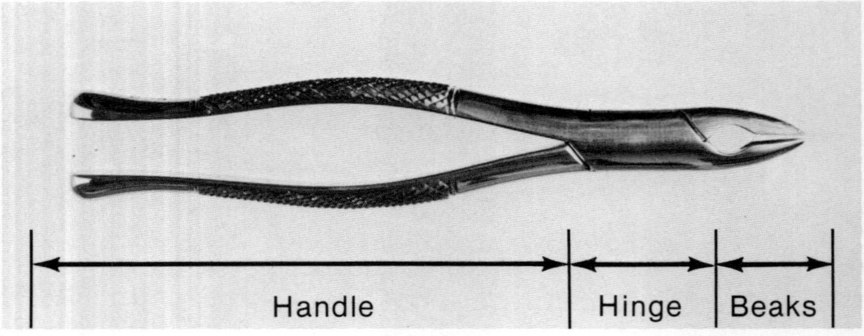

Figure I-1. Basic components of an extraction forceps.

- **Handle**

The handle of a forceps allows the instrument to be grasped in such a way as to deliver adequate leverage and pressure to the beaks. Handles for forceps used in the mandibular arch are designed either horizontally or vertically. The grasps for these two designs are shown in **Figure I-2.**

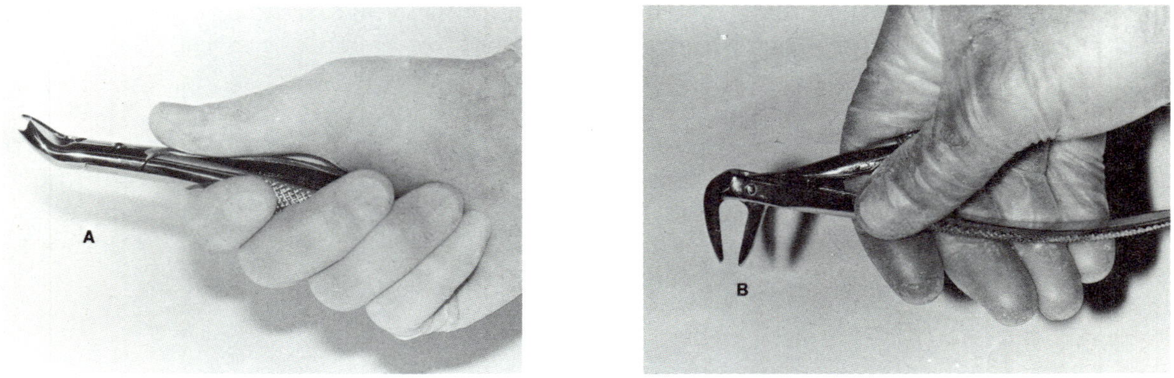

Figure I-2. Two basic methods for grasping forceps handles. A. A horizontal grasp is used with the American style forceps, such as the #90. B. Vertical grasp is used for the English or European style forceps, such as the #74 forceps.

The **horizontal-handled grasped** forceps are designed so that the forceps handle fits the palm of your hand such that the handles are horizontal to the floor when applied to teeth. They are grasped with the palm down for mandibular extractions or palm up for maxillary extractions when operating at a 7 to 9 o'clock right-handed position (3 to 5 o'clock for left handers). See **Figure I-3.**

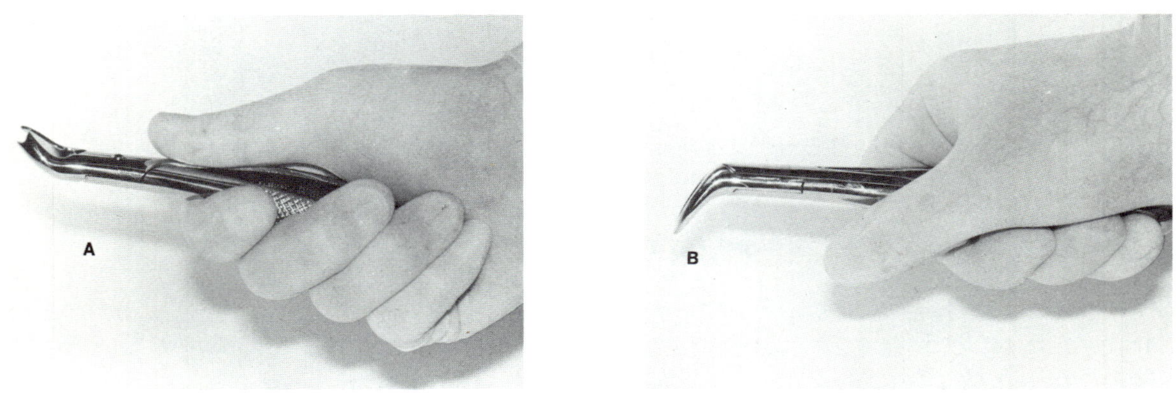

Figure I-3. Orientation of the palm of the hand when using grasping forceps for maxillary and mandibular extractions. A. Palm up for maxillary extractions. B. Palm down for mandibular extractions.

The handles of the **vertically grasped** English or European style forceps are designed to be held with the palm of the hand in a vertical plane for removal of mandibular teeth.

More leverage can be obtained with the **vertically grasped** English or European style forceps than with the horizontally grasped American style forceps. However, the greater leverage provided by the vertically grasped forceps can result in an increased frequency of root tip or coronal fracture if forces are not carefully controlled.

Forceps handles are also manufactured for right- or left-handed surgeons. Generally speaking, this does not become a major factor until you purchase your own equipment or request instruments for your clinic. You should specify which type you need when ordering these instruments.

Forceps handles are manufactured with many specialized shapes, three of which are shown in **Figure I-4**. Most dental faculty prefer to emphasize the use of straight- or droop-handled forceps believing these to be more versatile, thus requiring a fewer number of forceps. Institutional settings such as hospitals, large clinics, or group practices prefer to purchase instruments that can be used by many persons rather than to cater to specialized needs.

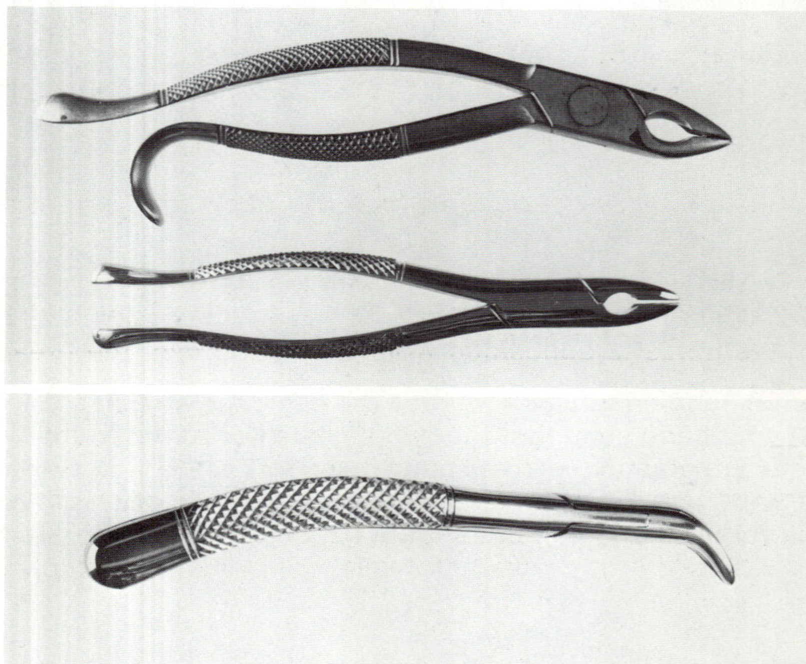

Figure I-4. Three varieties of forceps handle shapes. Straight or droop handles are preferred in most institutional settings.

STUDY EXERCISES — Forceps Handles

Forceps handles are designed to be held either HORIZONTALLY *as found in the American style or* VERTICALLY *as found in the English or European style. The English or European style provides more* LEVERAGE *; however, this advantage can lead to an increased incidence of* ROOT TIP OR CORONAL FRACTURE *if not carefully controlled, especially in the hands of a novice.*

The handle style preferred by most U. S. clinics or institutions is the (straight/curved) STRAIGHT *style. The reason for this is* BECAUSE THEY ARE MORE VERSATILE *.*

- **Hinge**

The hinge of a forceps acts to transfer and amplify the gripping force from the handle to the beaks. The hinge is oriented in the same plane as the handle.

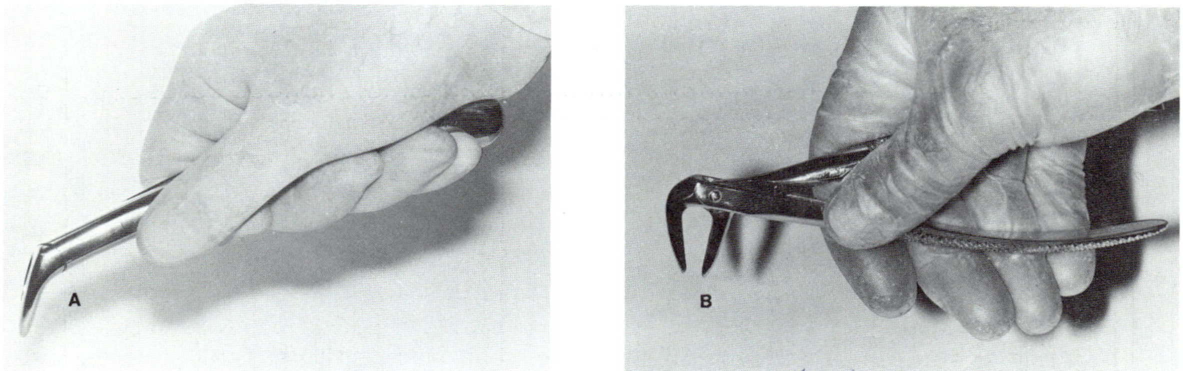

Figure I-5. Forceps hinges are in the same plane as their handles. A. #151 forceps with horizontal hinge and handle. B. A #74 forceps with a vertical hinge and handle.

From a functional point of view, most forceps hinges are satisfactorily designed. There are some considerations which should be discussed, including:

- **Danger to Soft Tissue**

  Occasionally, a hinge is designed which will allow inadvertent crush injuries to the lip.

- **Cleaning**

  The more the hinge is concealed from the naked eye, the greater the cleaning problem. The advent of ultrasonic cleaners removes most of this objection.

- **Lubrication**

  The greater the contact of metal, the greater the lubrication problem. It should be noted that rust tends to accumulate faster in hidden areas. Hinges may be lubricated with a silicone lubricant available from dental supply houses.

NOTE: You should always watch to see if your forceps is pinching tissue during an extraction procedure.

- **Beaks**

The beaks of an extraction forceps are designed on an anatomical basis. The beaks generally adapt to the tooth at a level near or below the cervical line of the tooth. The lower a beak grasps the tooth the less the risk of tooth fracture. In this functioning location, the beaks must adapt to conical, bifurcated, or trifurcated teeth. To accomplish this, the inner surfaces of most beaks are basically concave with additional projections for adaptation to furcations. This relationship is diagramed in **Figure I-6.**

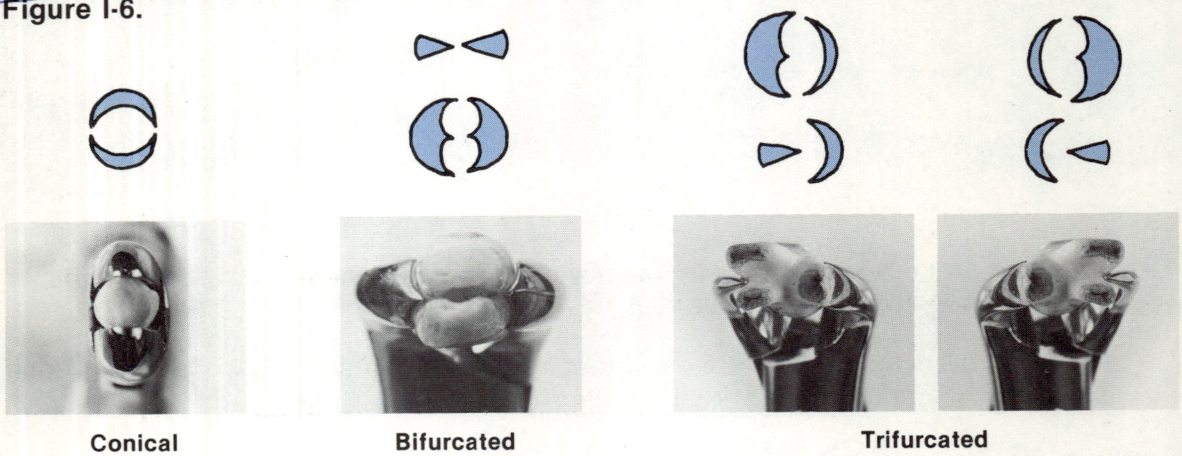

Figure I-6. Configuration of the inner surface of forceps beaks. Forceps designed for trifurcated molars are designed for either right or left sides.

Figure I-7 shows some typical ways forceps beaks adapt to specific tooth morphologies.

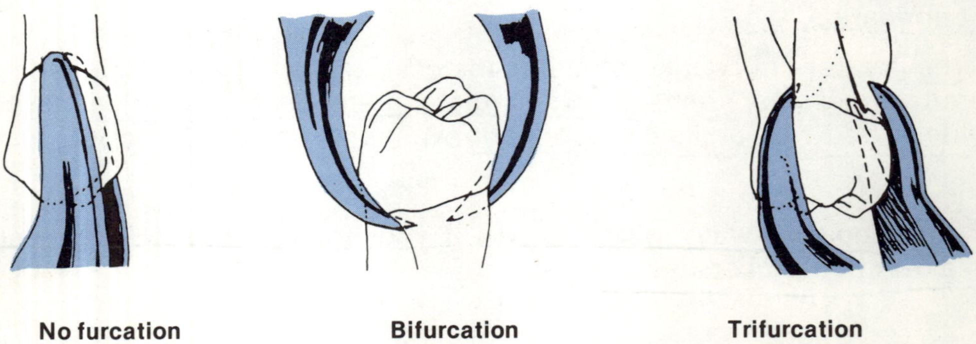

Figure I-7. Adaption of forceps beaks to various tooth morphologies.

Beak widths and adaptation to root and crown.

Most forceps beaks are designed to cradle crowns at or below the buccal and lingual height of contour and extend beyond the line angles just into the embrasures. If beaks are **too wide** they may damage adjacent teeth or provide an unstable grasp due to a one-point contact on hard enamel in the center of the beak (see **Figure I-8**). If beaks are too narrow for a specific crown the forceps also may be unstable because the sides of the beaks may not be able to grip hard enamel or root structure (see **Figure I-8**).

Beaks should adapt to the size of the roots. Beaks that are too large will not be able to migrate apically during an extraction because they will impinge on alveolar bone. Beaks that are too small may not grasp the root sufficiently. You should choose a beak design that best adapts to the size and shape of the tooth to be removed.

Figure I-8. The size of forceps beaks should adapt to the root contour of the tooth to be removed. A. Good adaptation. B. Poor adaptation of beaks in the root region.

While an experienced surgeon can compensate for discrepancies in forceps design, thus permitting more versatility for certain forceps, a novice is well advised to use forceps which are specifically designed for the anticipated surgery.

NOTE: Since there is such a great variation in the anatomy of teeth, what a forceps gains in universality it loses in specific anatomical adaption.

A novice would do well to choose a #89 for the extraction of an upper first molar instead of a #150 forceps (which might very well be used by the trained oral surgeon). It can be seen that the #89 is specifically designed so that one beak will enter the buccal trifurcation and the palatal beak will cradle the palatal root of an upper first molar. With sufficient pressure and correct adaptations, #89 forceps will adapt to the anatomy of the first molar and successfully lift it from its socket. On the other hand, one beak of the #150 forceps will slip part way into the buccal bifurcation, while the other beak is frustrated in its efforts to gain entry beneath the cervical line on the palatal aspect. Therefore, it is not as suitable for a maxillary molar extraction (see **Figure I-9**).

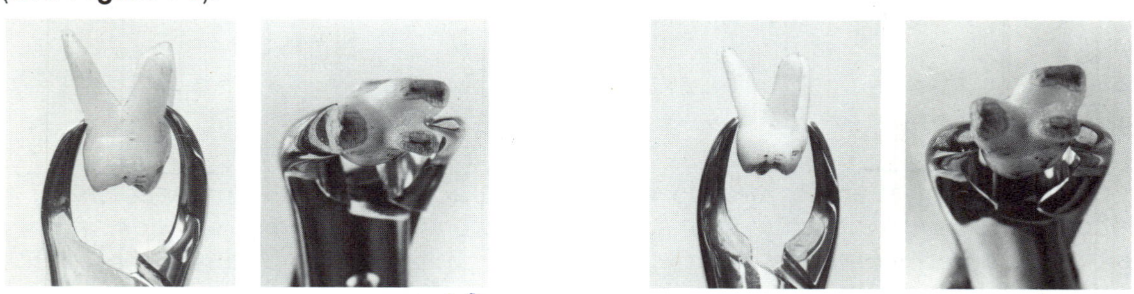

A. More efficient **B. Less efficient**

Figure I-9. Efficient and less efficient forceps adaption to a maxillary first molar. A. A #89 right maxillary molar forceps is designed to adapt to the trifurcated root structure. B. A #150-A forceps designed for maxillary pre-molars does not adapt as well to the trifurcated right maxillary first molar.

In general, the beaks of maxillary forceps are either parallel to the handle or are offset on the order of 45°. The beaks of the mandibular forceps are at about a right angle (perpendicular) to the handle (see **Figure I-10**). This difference in design facilitates adaption to teeth when the surgeon is positioned in front of or beside the patient.

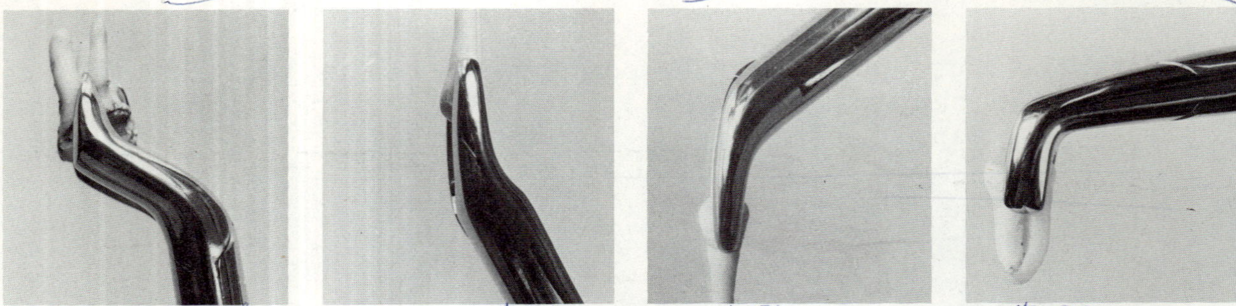

Figure I-10. Angulation of forceps beaks to the handle for maxillary and mandibular forceps. A. #88R. B. #150. C. #151. D. #222.

STUDY EXERCISES — Beaks

Forceps beaks are designed on an ____________ basis. They are designed to grasp the tooth at the ____________ level of the tooth. The lower a beak grasps a tooth the ____________ the risk of ____________ ____________.

Name the type of tooth morphology for which each of the following beak sketches is designed.

A B C

A. ____________
B. ____________
C. ____________

Beaks should be chosen to ____________ to specific tooth ____________ and ____________.

Answers

A. Maxillary molars B. Mandibular molars C. Incisors, canines and premolars

SPECIFIC FORCEPS

This discussion of specific forceps will be approached from the perspective of tooth morphology. We will primarily emphasize the anatomical design of forceps and include specific numbered examples. In practice you may use different numbers or encounter different numbering systems in other parts of the world. Through learning an anatomical approach you'll be able to quickly adapt to these changes.

Forceps for Extraction of Maxillary Teeth

Maxillary Anterior Teeth

Maxillary anterior teeth, including **incisors** and **canines,** generally have conical to triangular shaped roots. Forceps designed for extraction of these teeth include the following. (Extraction of canine teeth frequently involves surgical removal of buccal bone. See **Chapter 2, The Removal of Teeth.**)

☐ **#1**
☐ **#99-C**

These forceps are straight from handle to beak. They are designed to adapt to anterior teeth.

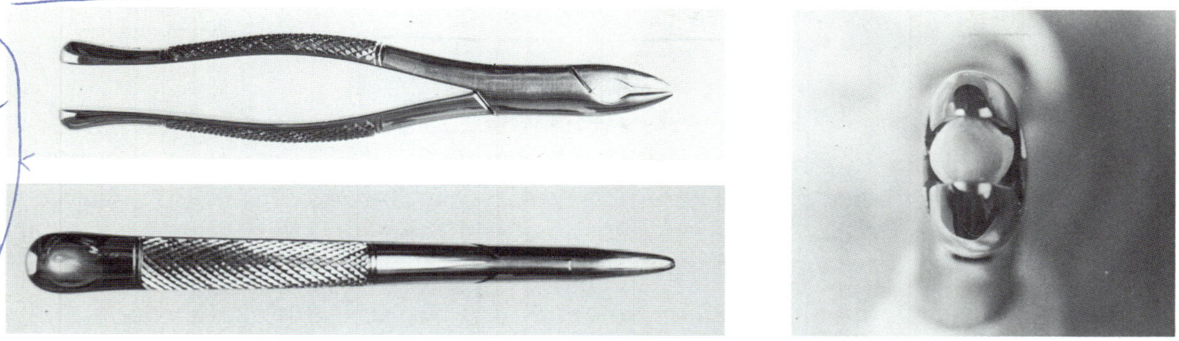

Figure I-11. A #1 or #99-C forceps is used for extraction of maxillary anterior teeth.

Maxillary incisors and canines are frequently removed using the #150 forceps; however, due to the angle of their beaks, they are a little more awkward to use for extraction of incisors.

Maxillary Premolars

Maxillary first premolars usually have a bifurcated root; however, the two roots lie in a buccal-lingual plane. Thus the root morphology resembles a conical root when considering forceps selection.

Maxillary second premolars generally have single conical roots; however, apical bifurcations are not uncommon.

☐ **#150**

Anatomically, these forceps are designed primarily for the premolar teeth. However, they are frequently used as "universal" forceps. They are not quite as effective as the #1 forceps for the extraction of the central incisor because of the curvature of the beaks. The beaks of a #150 forceps have a tendency to migrate towards the apex of an anterior tooth when proper apical forces are applied. This, of course, is a desirable attribute in a forceps.

These forceps are well suited for extraction of conically-shaped molars when the beaks are applied beneath the cervical line, but are poorly suited for the extraction of trifurcated molars, since the forceps beaks do not adapt closely to the molar crowns. They can also be used for maxillary root fragments or sectioned molars.

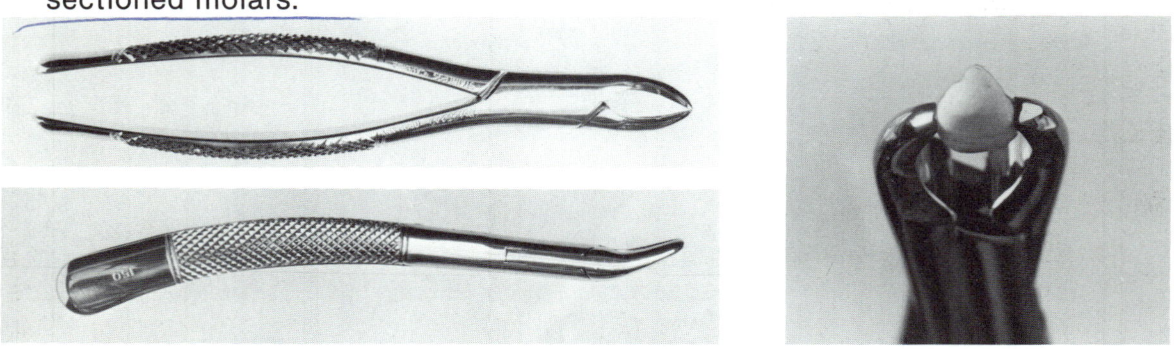

Figure I-12. A #150 forceps is designed for extraction of maxillary premolars and can be used for other maxillary teeth.

☐ #150-A

The #150-A forceps are specifically designed to conform to premolar crowns. They differ from the #150 in that their beaks are more parallel which permits better adaptation to premolar crowns, but poorer adaptation to maxillary anterior teeth. The #150-A does not tend to move apically as well as the #150 when force is applied to the handles.

First and Second Maxillary Molars

Maxillary first molars are the largest teeth and are usually trifurcated with a single palatal root and two buccal roots. **Maxillary second molars** are smaller and also have trifurcated roots, but to a lesser degree than the first molars. Occasionally second molars have nearly conical roots.

The important factor for forceps selection for extracting maxillary molars include selecting a forceps that will fit into the buccal furcation and at the same time grasp the palatal root firmly. You will need a pair of forceps for extracting maxillary molars; one for the right side and one for the left.

☐ #89 & 90

The #89 & 90 forceps are similar to the #88R & L with regard to application of the buccal prong; however, the palatal beak adapts to the palatal root rather than entering the furcations.

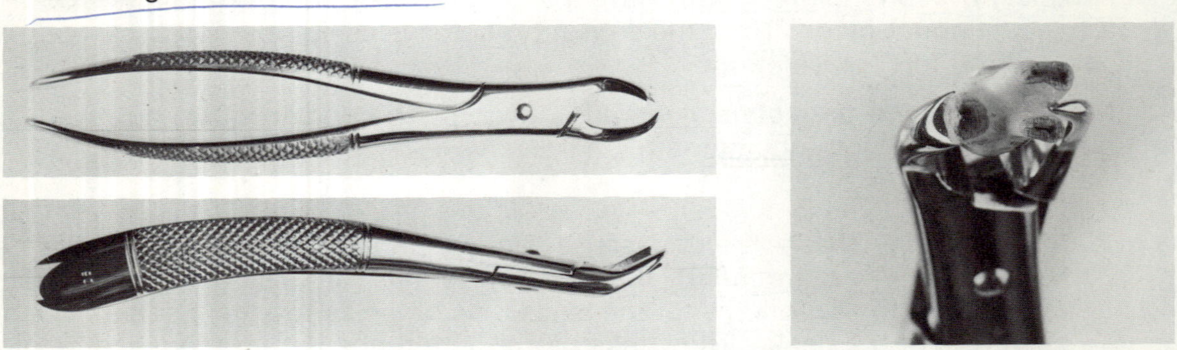

Figure I-13. The #89 & 90 forceps.

☐ #88R & L

The #88R & L forceps have a three-pronged beak and are often referred to as "upper cowhorn" forceps. The two palatal prongs slide to either side of the palatal root while the buccal prong enters the furcation between the mesio-buccal and distal-buccal roots. Reckless use of these forceps can result in alveolar fracture, crushing of gingival tissue, or damage to adjacent teeth.

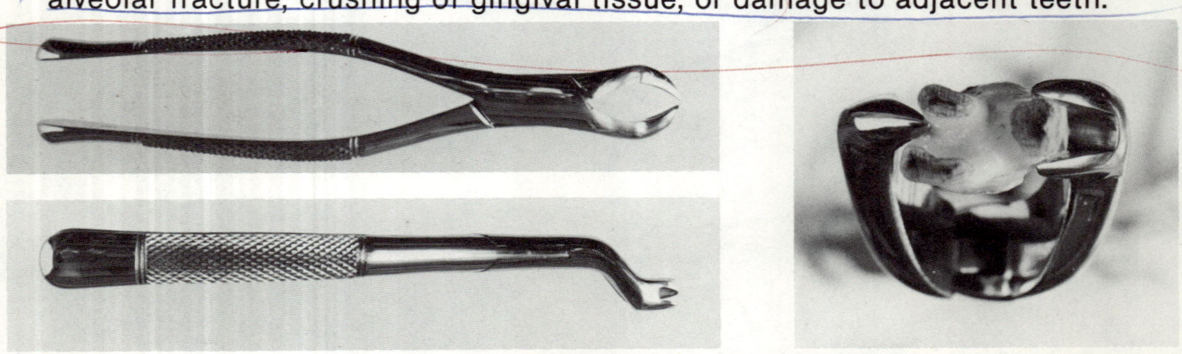

Figure I-14. The #88R & L forceps.

Both #89 & 90 and #88R & L apply their force below the cervical line and are better suited for removing teeth which have extensive coronal caries or large coronal restorations.

□ #53R & L

The 53R & L are designed to extract trifurcated maxillary first and second molars. Their specific anatomical features are a pointed buccal beak which is also grooved to fit the buccal trifurcation. This forceps provides very good adaptation to the molar crown, but should not be used when caries are extensive, when a very large amalgam restoration is present, or in some cases when endodontic treatment has rendered the crown brittle.

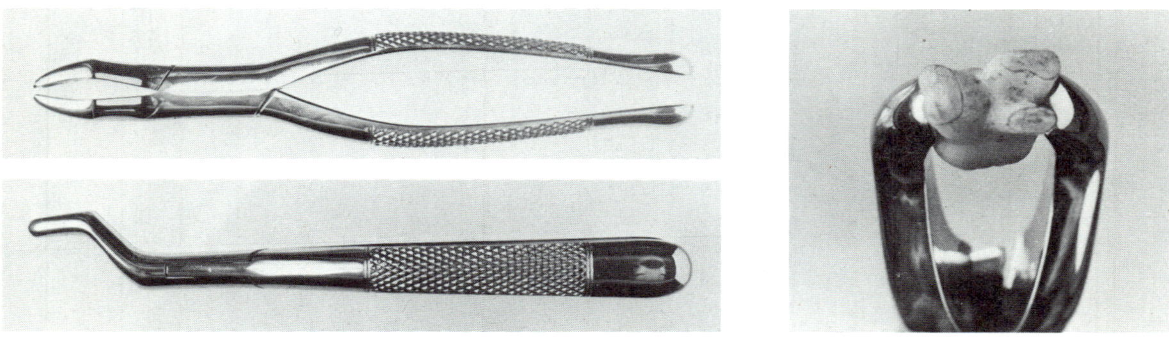

Figure I-15. The #53R & L forceps are designed for maxillary molars with reduced trifurcations. They should be used when the crown is intact.

Erupted Maxillary Third Molars

Most maxillary third molars have conical roots; however, bifurcations or trifurcations are also found. Most maxillary third molars can be removed easily, but occasionally you will need maximum help provided through a well-designed forceps.

□ **#210-S**

This forceps is designed especially for the extraction of the erupted maxillary third molar and is bayonet-shaped. Its beaks are shorter than the other similar-appearing forceps such as the #53 because the clinical crown of the third molar is usually shorter.

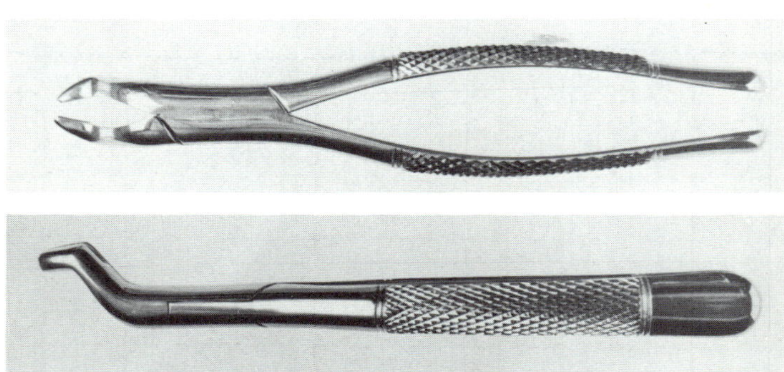

Figure I-16. The #210-S forceps is designed for erupted maxillary third molars.

Maxillary Root Fragments

Root fragments remaining as a result of extensive caries can be difficult to extract with forceps designed to grasp intact teeth. Root fragments are generally narrow and conical in shape.

☐ **#286**

The #286 forceps is bayonet-shaped and is primarily designed for the extraction of maxillary root tips. They are sometimes used for the extraction of maxillary premolars especially when premolars are very small. The beaks of the #286 are long and slender.

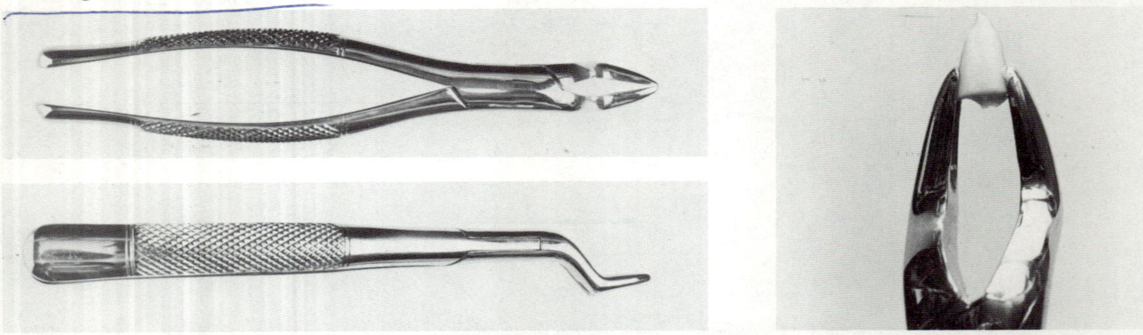

Figure I-17. The #286 forceps is designed for removal of maxillary root tips.

Forceps for extraction of primary teeth

☐ **#150-S**

The #150-S is a smaller version of the #150 forceps. This forceps adapts reasonably well to all primary teeth in the maxillary arch.

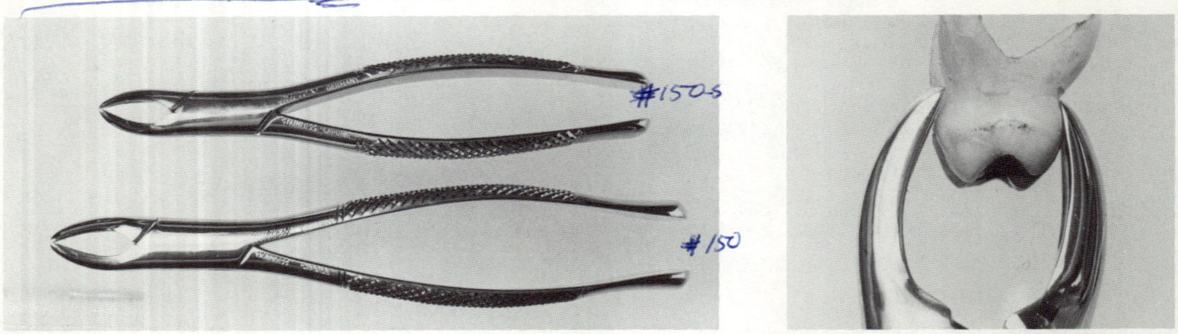

Figure I-18. The #150-S is designed for extraction of primary maxillary teeth. The above photographs show the relative size comparison between the #150-S (top) and the #150 (bottom).

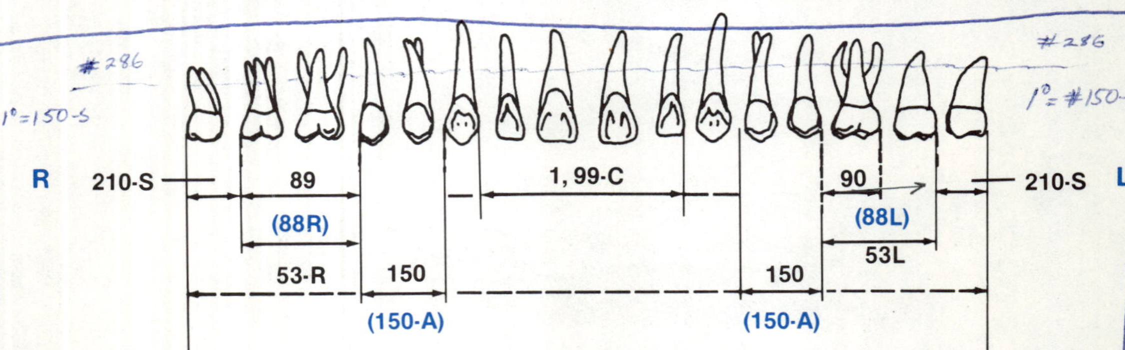

Figure I-19. Summary diagram for selection of maxillary forceps.

STUDY EXERCISES

Complete the following diagram stating the specific forceps number to be used in each area.

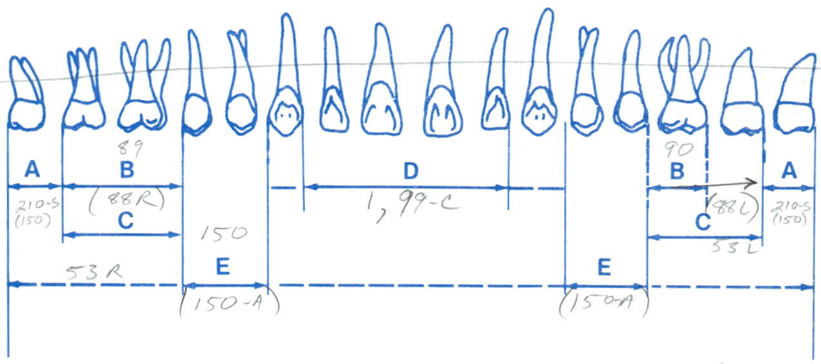

The # 150 forceps is frequently used as an upper "universal." This forceps adapts well to maxillary PREMOLAR teeth but does not adapt well to trifurcated maxillary MOLARS .

If the crown of a maxillary first molar is seriously damaged by caries you would best select a # 89, 90 or 88 R, 88 L forceps. If the crown is not damaged you could select a # 53R, 53L forceps.

The # 88R, 88L forceps is extremely efficient and if used in a reckless fashion can result in serious complications.

The forceps you should select for removal of maxillary root fragments is the # 286 .

Maxillary primary teeth are removed using a # 150-S forceps.

ANSWERS TO FORCEPS SELECTION CHART

A. #210-S. B. #89-90. C. #53 R&L. D. #1 or #99-C. E. #150.

Forceps for Extraction of Mandibular Teeth

Mandibular Anterior and Premolar Teeth

Mandibular incisors have single roots that are flattened in the mesial-distal direction. Mandibular canines have the longest roots in the entire arch and generally require surgical removal of bone as described in **Chapter 2, The Removal of Teeth**. Mandibular premolars are generally single rooted and can be removed with the same forceps as used for other mandibular anterior teeth.

☐ **#74, 74-N, and 74-extra-N.**

These forceps are very well designed for the extraction of the mandibular incisor teeth and mandibular root tips. They are of the vertical English or European style. #74-N has narrower beaks and the #74-extra-N has even narrower beaks. Because of the vertical handle design, there is a tendency for the novice to break teeth with this forceps. The expert prevents this by continually seating the forceps beaks during the extraction, thus placing the fulcrum of extraction lower on the root in an area which can bear more stress. There are numerous forceps with a different numerical designation which are almost identical to the #74. In general, they are all satisfactory.

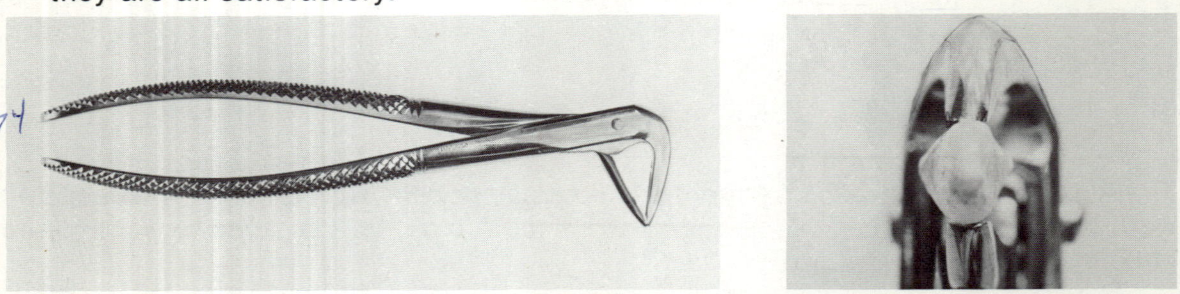

Figure I-20. The #74 English or European style forceps is designed for mandibular anterior teeth. Narrow and extra-narrow models are also available.

☐ **#151 and 151-A**

The #151 is primarily used for removal of mandibular premolar teeth and some root tips. However, they are used very successfully for the extraction of all mandibular premolars and anterior teeth, as well as erupted third molars. These forceps are often referred to as lower "universal" forceps. Like the #150-A, the #151-A is designed to grasp mandibular premolar crowns, but does not adapt as well as the #151 to other mandibular teeth.

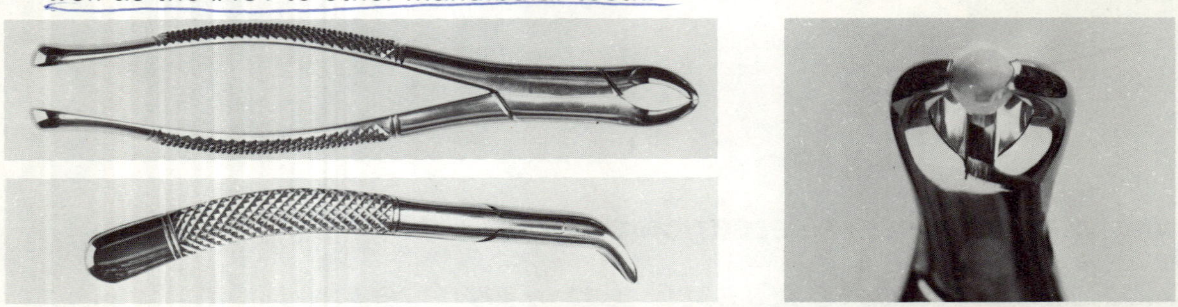

Figure I-21. The #151 forceps is designed for the removal of mandibular premolars, but can also be used for other mandibular teeth..

The **#203** is similar to the #150 and #150-A; however, the beaks are thinner, allowing better adaptation to the crowns of incisors and root tips.

Mandibular Molars

Mandibular first molars are bifurcated in the mesial-distal direction creating a buccal and lingual furcation. Mandibular second molars are usually bifurcated to a lesser extent than first molars. Frequently they have conical roots without furcations.

Some mandibular forceps are designed to take advantage of this bifurcation; however, when the tooth is not bifurcated other forceps must be used.

☐ #23 (Cowhorn)

The #23 or "cowhorn" forceps was first designed in 1884, and has been the most popular mandibular molar forceps since that time. The beaks are designed to enter the bifurcation of the mandibular molar. Since it is imperative that the beaks do enter the bifurcation, this forceps must be applied even more carefully than the others. Once it is properly adapted to the tooth it can, in some instances, extract a molar teeth simply by means of "squeezing it out of the socket." This squeezing effect is achieved when the beaks of the forceps are squeezed between the buccal and lingual plates of bone and the tooth.

While this squeezing action is a part of the extraction of the mandibular molar teeth, it is ordinarily used in conjunction with some buccal-lingual movement. (See **Chapter 2, The Removal of Teeth.**)

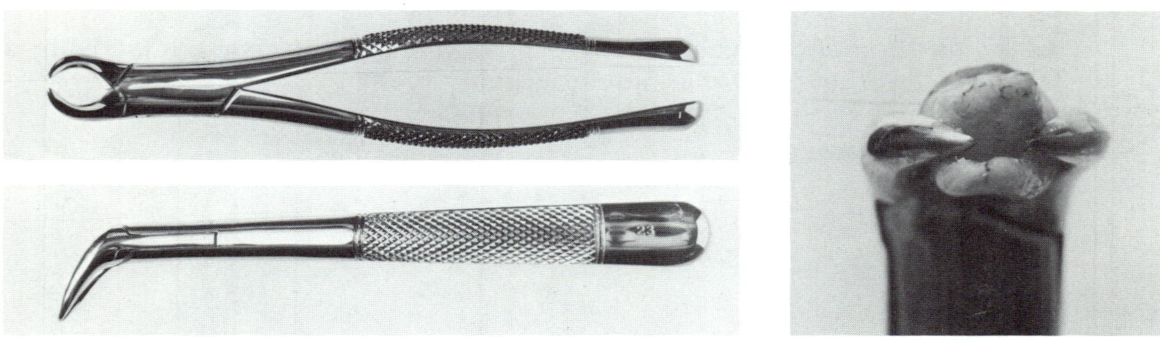

Figure I-22. The #23 forceps is designed for bifurcated mandibular molars with divergent roots.

☐ #17

The #17 forceps are designed to extract bifurcated mandibular first and second molars. Their specific anatomical features are pointed beaks which also are grooved on the internal surface. This allows the beaks to adapt to the crown, and also to enter the bifurcation.

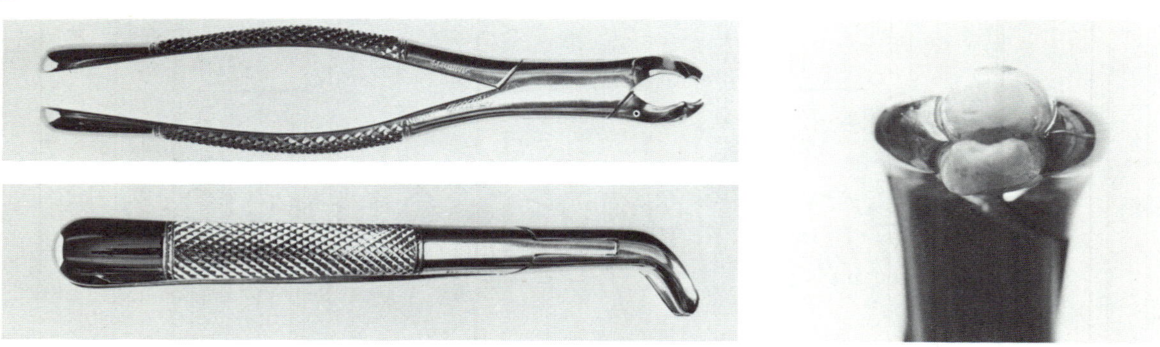

Figure I-23. The #17 forceps is designed for mandibular molars with convergent roots.

Erupted Mandibular Third Molars

□ **#222**

The #222 is designed especially to extract erupted mandibular third molars. The beaks are almost 90° to the handle allowing easy access to the third molar region.

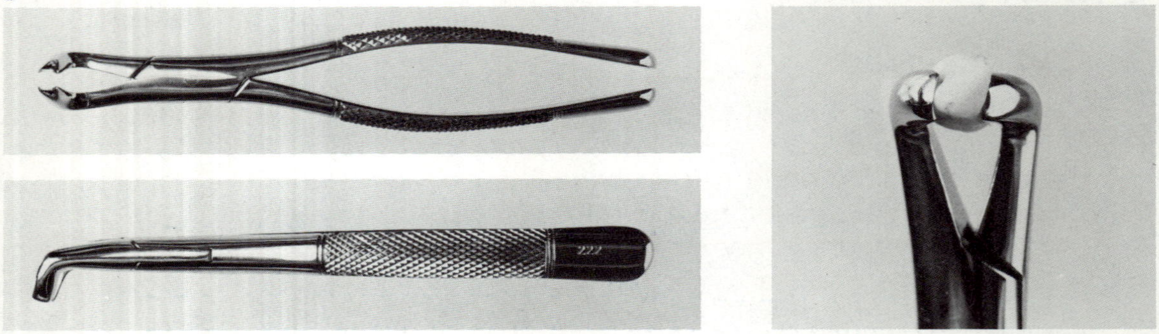

Figure I-24. The #222 forceps is designed for erupted mandibular third molars.

Primary Mandibular Teeth

□ **#151-S**

As the name implies, this is a scaled-down version of the #151. It is ideally suited for the extraction of all mandibular primary teeth.

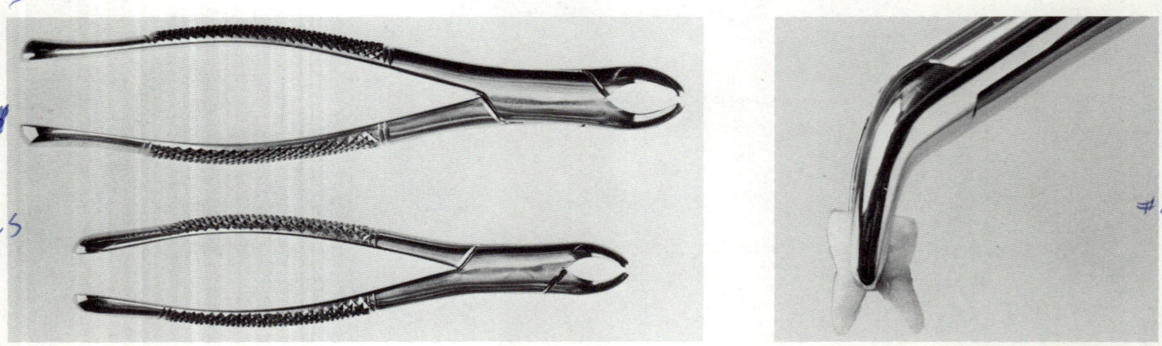

Figure I-25. The #151-S is designed for extraction of primary mandibular teeth.

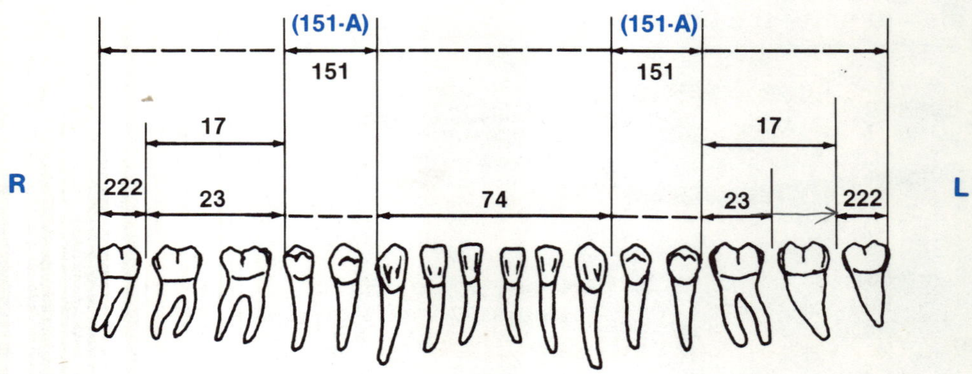

Figure I-26. Summary diagram for selection of forceps for removing mandibular teeth.

STUDY EXERCISES — Forceps for Mandibular Extractions

Complete the following diagram stating the specific forceps number to be used in each area.

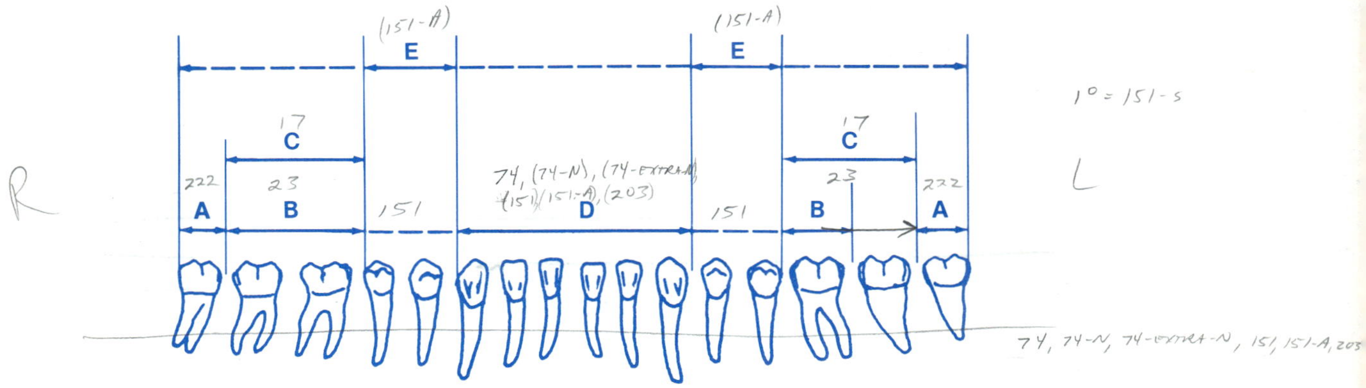

The # 74 forceps is available in a variety of widths and is used for removal of mandibular incisors, canines, and premolars. The narrower versions such as # 74-N and # 74-EXTRA-N are frequently of use when MANDIBULAR ANTERIORS, (ROOT TIPS) are small. The #203 can also be used for (MANDIBULAR ANTERIORS), ROOT TIPS.

The # 151 forceps is frequently referred to as the lower " UNIVERSAL ." It is designed primarily for mandibular PREMOLARS, ROOT TIPS . You will find the beaks too large to use on MANDIBULAR ANTERIORS , and somewhat small to use on MAND. MOLARS .

The # 151-A is similar to the #151; however, it does not adapt as well to MAND. ANTERIORS or MAND. MOLARS .

The # 23 forceps is used for bifurcated mandibular first molars. A better choice for fused rooted mandibular second molars would be the # 17 or # 151 forceps.

The # 222 forceps is used for conical rooted mandibular third molars.

Mandibular root tips are removed with the # 74 (74-N), (74-EXTRA-N) or # 151 (151-A), (203) forceps.

Mandibular primary teeth are removed with the # 151-S forceps.

ANSWERS TO FORCEPS SELECTION CHART

A. #222. B. #23. C. #17. D. #74. E. #151.

Unit II

ELEVATORS

Introduction
Components of an Elevator
Use of Elevators
- Displacement
- Lever action
- Wheel and axle

Commonly Used Elevators
- #30 & 31 (Cryer)
- #41 (Crane pick)
- #73 & 74 Miller
- Potts
- #34-S & 46
- #301, 302, 303

Apex elevators (Root picks)

PRETEST

- *Answer each question by circling the correct answer.*
- *If all questions are answered correctly, proceed to Unit III, page 39.*
- *If you do not answer all questions correctly, read and study the content of this Unit.*
- *The numbers in parentheses at the end of each question refer to the specific objective number from which this question was derived.*

Questions:

_______ 1. *The three basic components of an elevator are (01-02-01):*
- *a. Beak, shank, hinge*
- *b. Handle, hinge & tip*
- *c. Handle, shank & tip*
- *d. Handle, shank & beak*
- *e. Handle, hinge & blade*

_______ 2. *The two basic types of elevators are (01-02-02):*
- *a. Inclined beak & displacement*
- *b. Inclined plane & lever*
- *c. Inclined plane and wheel & axle*
- *d. Inclined beak and wheel & axle*
- *e. None of the above*

_______ 3. *The three basic ways elevators are used are (01-02-03):*
- *a. Displacement, lever action, and wheel & axle*
- *b. Displacement, wheel & axle, and traction*
- *c. Rotation, traction, and wheel & axle*
- *d. All of the above (a, b, & c are correct)*
- *e. None of the above*

_______ 4. *The illustration shows which type of elevator action (01-02-03):*
- *a. Displacement*
- *b. Lever action*
- *c. Wheel & axle*
- *d. Traction*
- *e. None of the above*

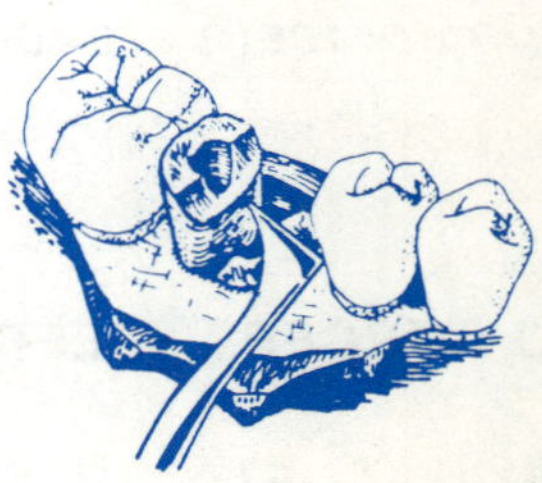

________ 5. *The illustration shows which type of elevator action (01-02-03):*

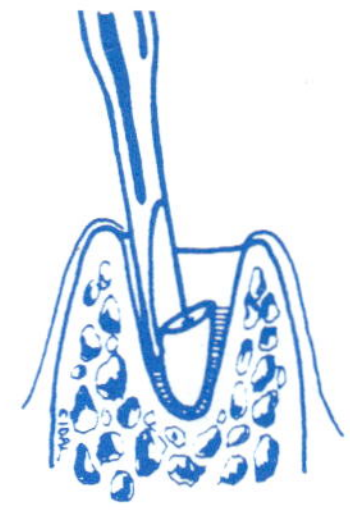

- *(a) Displacement*
- *b. Lever*
- *c. Wheel & axle*
- *d. Traction*
- *e. None of the above*

Which of the following elevators would be used in each of the following situations (use letter code from choices at right) (01-02-04):

B #41 (Crane pick) 6. *Used with purchase point and fulcrum on buccal bone (01-02-04-b)*

E Apex elevators 7. *Used for removing very small root tips (01-02-04-g)*

A #30-31 (Cryer) 8. *Used primarily for removing roots when there is an adjacent empty socket (01-02-04-a)*

C #34-S or #46 9. *Used for removing larger root fragments by displacement effect (01-02-04-e)*

D #301 10. *Used for removing small root tips and occasionally for beginning luxation of teeth when larger elevator is too large. (01-02-04-f)*

Choices

- *a. #30 - 31 (Cryer)*
- *b. #41 (Crane pick)*
- *c. #34-S or #46*
- *d. #301*
- *e. Apex elevators*

Identify each of the following elevators from the photographs of their blades or tips.

________ 11. *(01-02-05-a)*

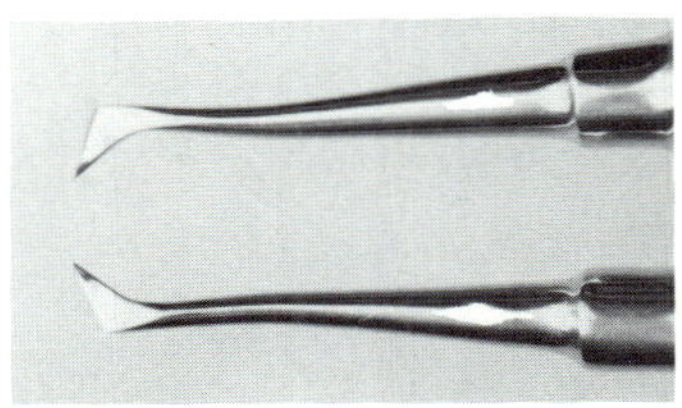

- *a. #301*
- *b. #34-S*
- *c. #73 - 74*
- *(d) #30 - 31* (Cryer)
- *e. #41*

________ 12. *(01-02-05-b)*

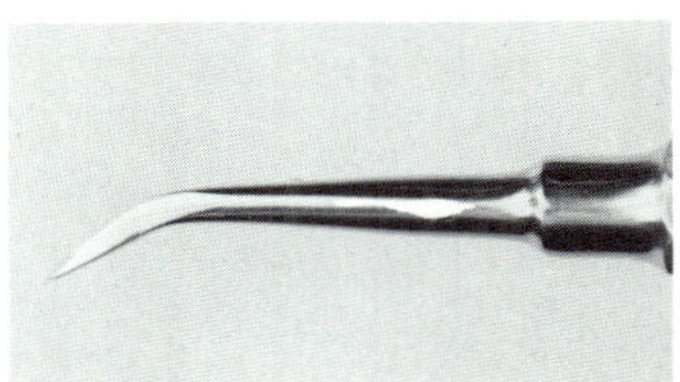

- *a. #301*
- *b. #34-S*
- *(c) #41* (Crane pick)
- *d. Potts*
- *e. Apex elevator*

________ 13. *(01-02-05-c)*

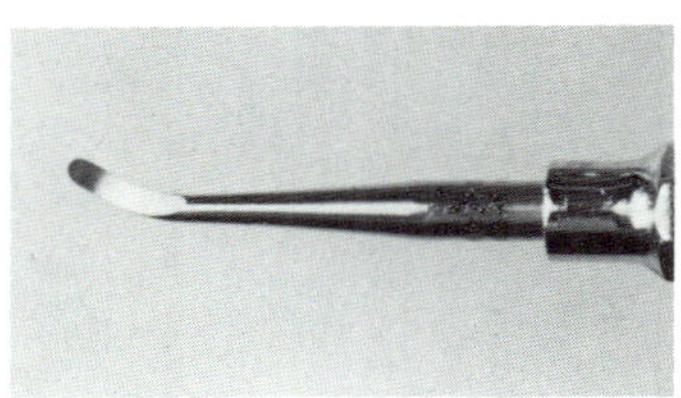

- *(a) #73 - 74 or Potts* (Miller)
- *b. #41*
- *c. #301*
- *d. #46*
- *e. #30 - 31*

_______ 14. (01-02-05-e)

a. #301
b. #41
c. #46 or 34-S
d. Apex elevator
e. #30 - 31

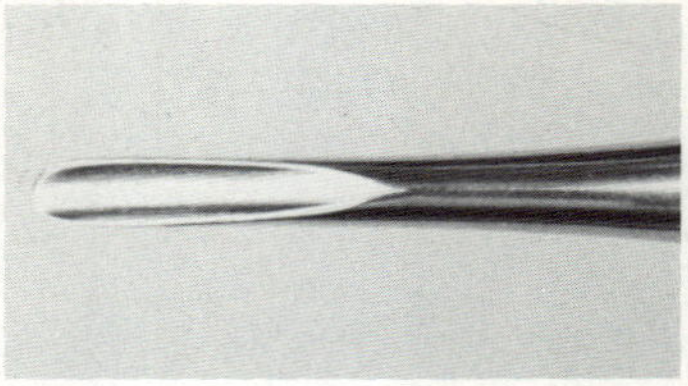

_______ 15. (01-02-05-f)

a. #34-S
b. #301
c. #41
d. #73 - 74 Miller
e. Apex elevator

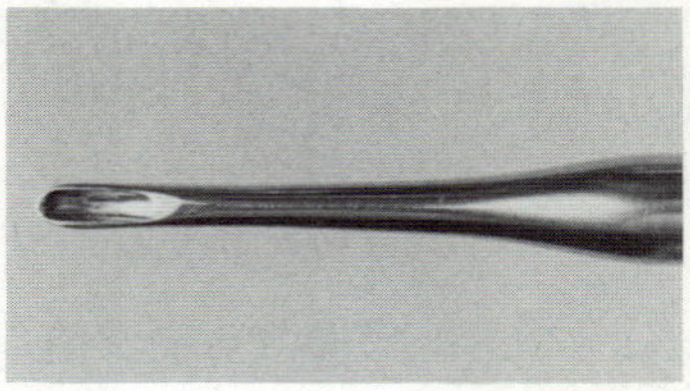

_______ 16. (01-02-05-g)

a. #46
b. #41
c. #73 - 74
d. #30 - 31
e. Apex elevator

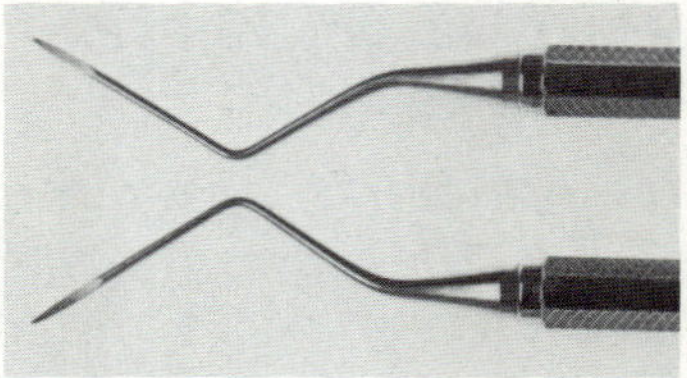

Answers

1.	c	5.	a	9.	c	13.	a
2.	c	6.	b	10.	d	14.	c
3.	a	7.	e	11.	d	15.	b
4.	c	8.	a	12.	c	16.	e

Unit II

ELEVATORS

INTRODUCTION

Elevators are a valuable aid to the extraction of teeth. Elevators are used to luxate (loosen) teeth or portions of teeth such as sectioned roots or fractured root tips. Some surgeons can remove most teeth with the use of elevators alone. While we do not advocate this for the novice, the use of elevators is an essential component to your surgical training.

Components of an Elevator

The basic components of an elevator are:

- Handle
- Shank
- Blade (or Tip)

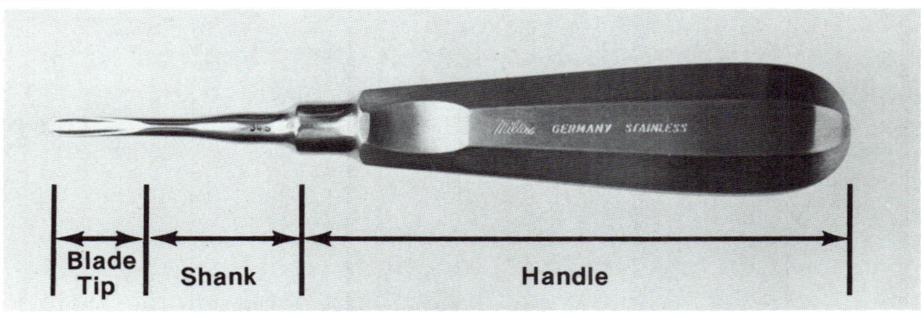

Figure II-1. Component parts of an elevator.

- **Handle**

  The handle of elevators is generally of substantial size so that it can be firmly grasped and held in control while in use. Elevators can inflict considerable damage if not used with controlled forces, especially the "T" bar handles as shown in **Figure II-1 (see Chapter 4, Surgical Complications)**.

- **Shank**

  The shank of an elevator should be strong to withstand the forces of action.

- **Blade or Tip**

  The portion of an elevator used to contact teeth is called the blade or tip, depending upon the type of elevator.

STUDY EXERCISE

The basic components of an elevator are the HANDLE, SHANK *and* BLADE *or* TIP.

Elevators are designed in two basic types:

- Inclined plane
- Wheel and axle

Use of Elevators

Elevators are used in three basic ways:

- Displacement (inclined plane)
- Lever action
- Wheel and axle

- **Displacement** of root tips by insertion into the periodontal ligament space. This action will frequently dislodge the root tip.

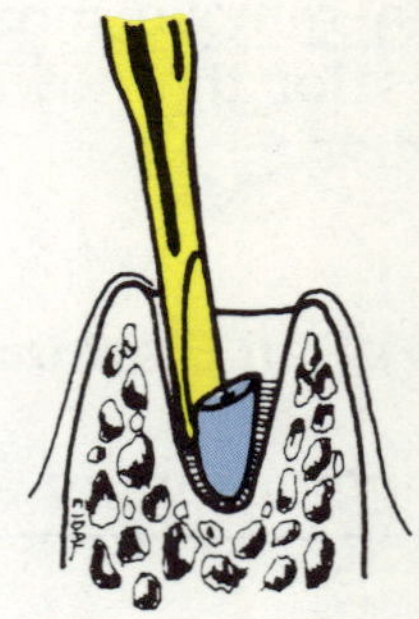

Figure II-2. Use of a shoehorn elevator for displacement of a root tip.

NOTE: You should not use this technique for removing root tips that are in close proximity to the maxillary sinus. You may displace the root tip into the sinus or create an oral-antral communication should the elevator slip past the root tip. (See **Chapter 4, Surgical Complications**.)

- **Lever action** is used for prying a tooth root tip from its socket. In this application the elevator engages the tooth through a **purchase point** (which is a groove or hole in the tooth placed with a bur) or through gripping the tooth with the edge of the blade and, using bone as a fulcrum, lifts the tooth from the socket when the handle is depressed.

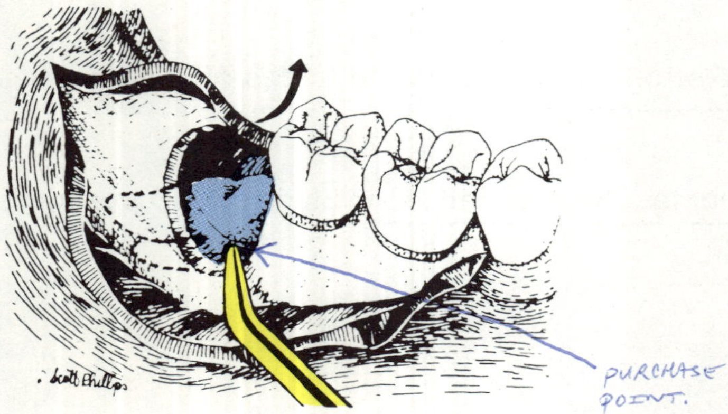

Figure II-3. Use of a #41 elevator to pry tooth out of socket.

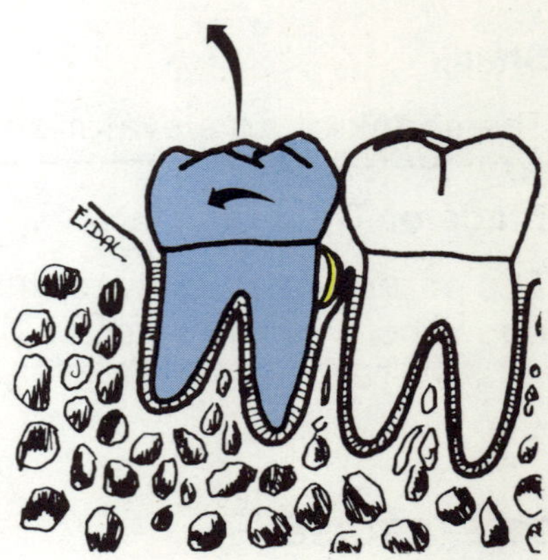

Figure II-4. Use of #46 elevator to luxate or loosen tooth.

- **Wheel and axle** action is produced when the elevator engages a purchase point and, using bone as a fulcrum, the elevator handle is rotated. This rotation is transmitted to the tip of the elevator and the tooth or root is displaced laterally to the line of the shaft.

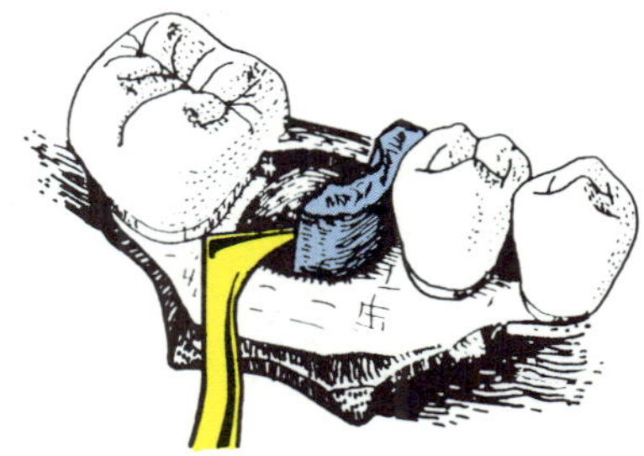

Figure II-5. Use of a #30 & 31 elevator rotating against buccal bone to push root tip from socket.

The two basic types of elevators are: 1) ______________________ *and 2)* ______________ *and* ______________ *.*

Elevators are used in three basic ways: 1) ______________________ *, 2)* ______________ ______________ *, and 3)* ______________ *.*

Commonly Used Elevators

The following elevators are commonly used. By no means have we tried to discuss the wide variety of available elevators. As with forceps, we've tried to select those which will be adequate for your basic instruction. You may find additional elevators that you prefer as you progress with your training. As part of the description of each elevator we will describe the manner in which it is used. Many are used in a combination of both lever and wheel and axle actions.

☐ **#30 & 31 (Cryer)**

This pair of elevators functions primarily by the wheel and axle method as demonstrated in **Figure II-5**. They can function with or without the use of a purchase point.

These elevators are used primarily to remove roots when there is an adjacent empty socket. The best example is the mandibular first molar area after the distal root has been extracted (see **Chapter 2, The Removal of Teeth**). The fulcrum will be placed on the buccal plate of bone, the sharp point of this elevator is sunk into the cementum of the mesial root, and the root is drawn out of the socket. Since the successful use of this elevator depends upon the sharpness of the tip, it is necessary to emphasize that this elevator must be sharpened at regular intervals. (See **Chapter 6, Assessment of and Surgery for the Impacted Mandibular Third Molar**, for examples of use of these instruments.) See **Figure II-5** for illustration of use.

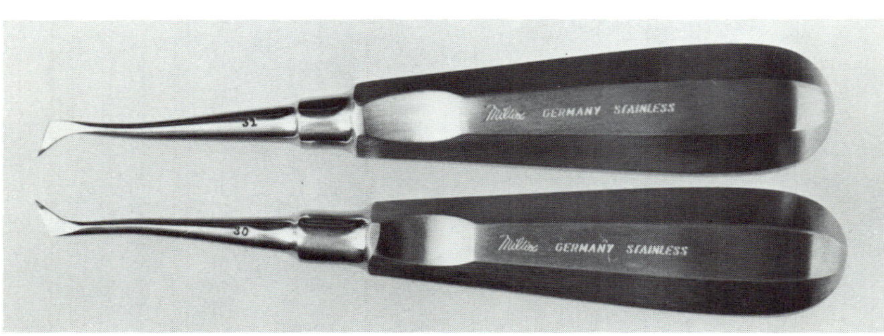

Figure II-6. The #30 & 31 (Cryer) elevators.

☐ #41 (Crane Pick)

The #41 or Crane pick is one of the handiest and also one of the MOST DANGEROUS elevators to be found. It is used primarily as a "wheel and axle" elevator. In other words, the fulcrum is placed on the buccal bone and its sharp point is buried into the cementum of the root and an attempt is made to drag the root out. It should be pointed out that no attempt should be made to extract a tooth with any elevator unless the root has a clear unobstructed path of exit. The use of force to bypass an obstruction of bone will either fracture the bone or fracture the tooth.

The #41 elevator is usually used with a purchase point, which is a hole placed in the root by means of a bur. Ideally, the hole should be at least 3 mm apical to the CEJ and at least 3 mm deep, in order to achieve effective elevation without breaking tooth structure. Use of this elevator is shown in **Figure II-3**.

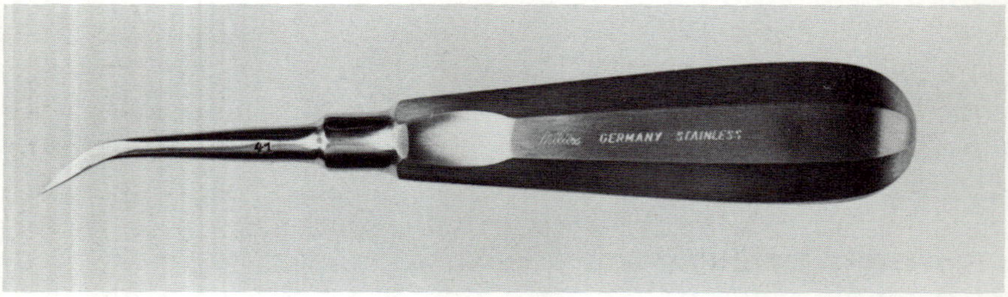

Figure II-7. The #41 (Crane pick) elevator.

☐ #73 & 74 (Miller)
☐ Potts elevators

The #73 & 74 Miller and the Potts elevators are designed for removing impacted maxillary third molars. The Potts elevators have "T"-bar handles which can deliver more force. They are NOT used as effectively when the maxillary third molar is erupted. The elevator blade is placed at the mesial buccal of the tooth at the level of the cervical line. It is forced toward the palate and at the same time the tooth is elevated distally. The elevator is used as a cork screw, i.e., in one movement the elevator is pushed palatally, superiorly, and distally. The third molar will elevate with ease if there is not excessive bony obstruction and if the roots are not unduly curved or divergent.

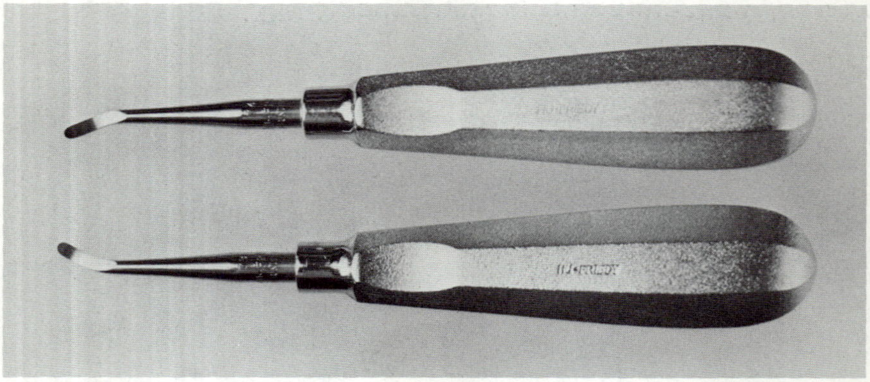

Figure II-8. The #73 & 74 Miller elevators

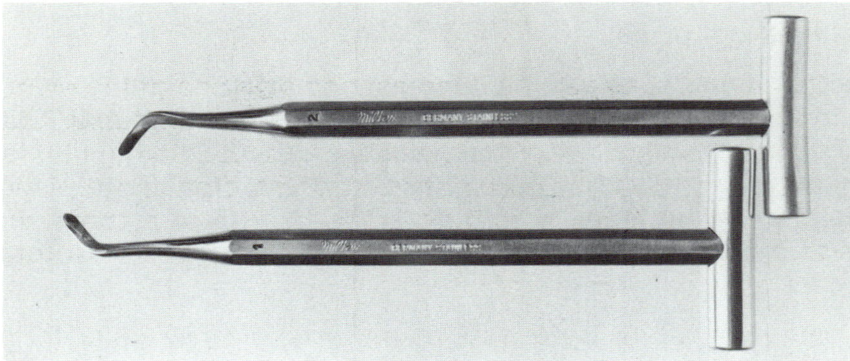

Figure II-9. Potts elevators.

T-BAR HANDLES.

□ #34-S and #46 (Large shoehorn, straight elevators)

The #34-S and #46 elevators are probably the most commonly used elevators, and are used in the extraction of almost every tooth. Their main use, however, is the removal of single roots by their displacement effect. The elevator, in an attempt to displace the tooth, is placed into the periodontal ligament space parallel to the tooth. Since a rather firm apical pressure is used for this elevator, it is important to grasp the elevator properly so it will not slip with an undue force. Use of these elevators is shown in **Figures II-2 and II-4**.

The #34-S is wider than the #46; therefore it is more useful on larger teeth.

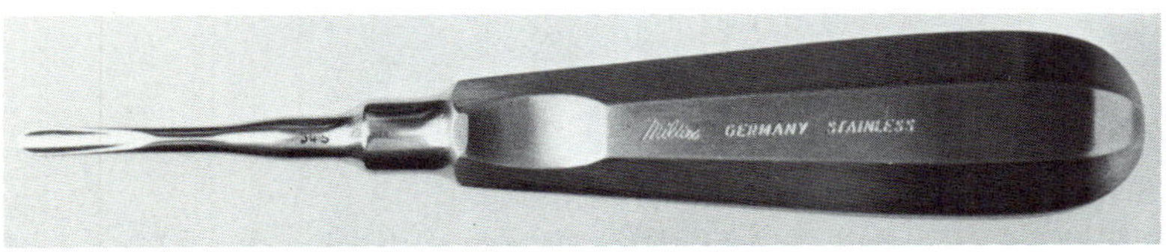

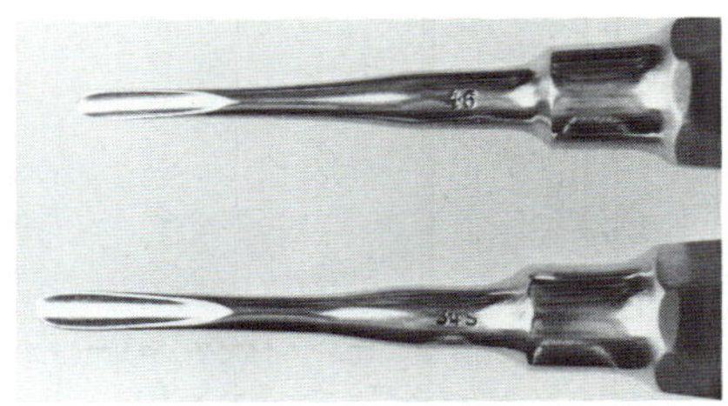

Figure II-10. The #34-S and #46 elevators.

□ #301, 302, 303

This series is an inclined plane elevator which is used similarly to the #34-S and #46, but for smaller roots. They are not "wheel and axle" elevators and are usually used either to tease out roots or to displace them by applying the force parallel to the surface of the root. Unsuccessful elevation with these instruments is usually due to an obstruction. In this event, the surgeon should not resort to more force, but should remove the obstruction. Often in the case of a high root fracture or if the root tip is tiny, the root tip is already somewhat loosened. Frequently when attempting to luxate teeth you can gain enough access with these smaller elevators, then progress to the #34-S or #46.

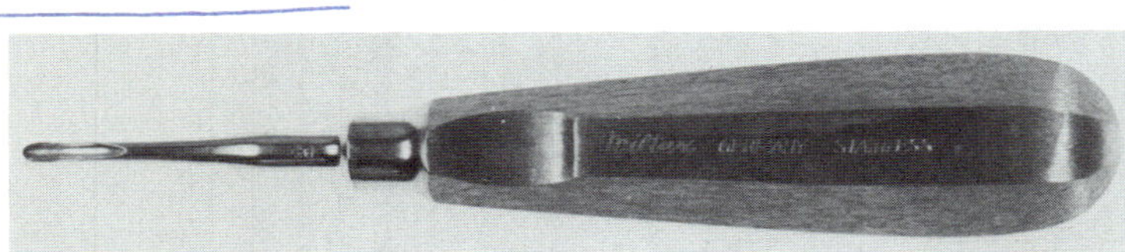

Figure II-11. The #301 elevator.

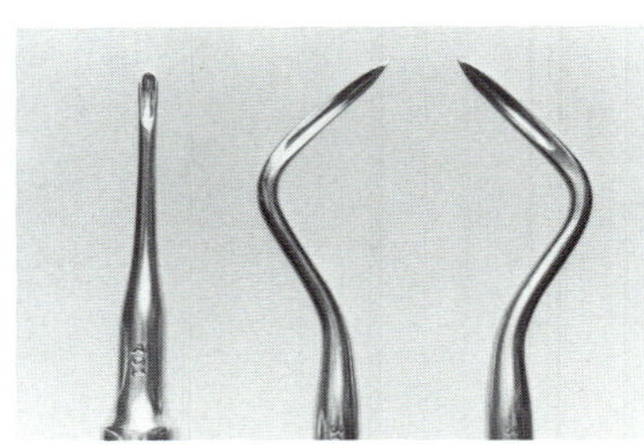

Figure II-12. Close-up view of the blades of the #301, 302 & 303.

□ Apex elevators (Root picks)

Apex elevators have either a straight shank or are angled. They are available in sets of variable sizes; however, the larger sizes are bulky and offer very little advantages over the #301. **Very small** apex elevators are essential instruments in the removal of small detached root tips, especially if the root tip is slightly loose. These are delicate instruments and cannot be used with appreciable force.

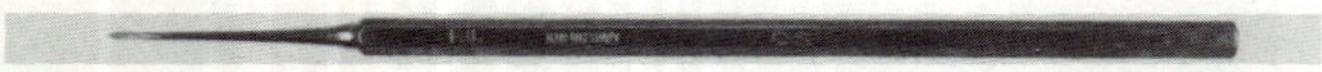

Straight shank.

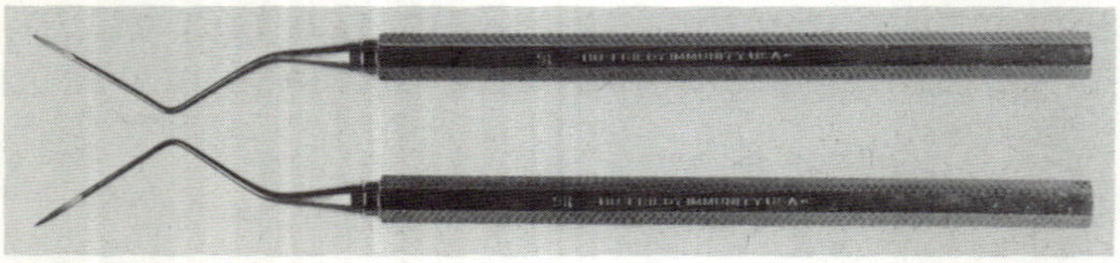

Angled shank.

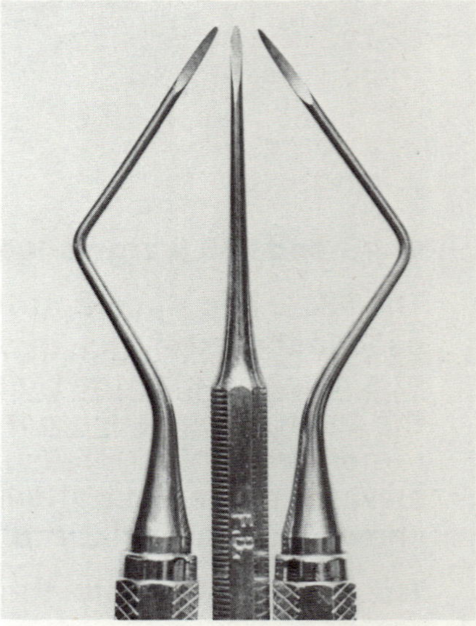

Figure II-13. Apex elevators (root picks), angled shanks for removal of detached root tips.

They are used individually or in pairs (chopsticks). When used individually, the sharp end is placed in the PDL space and the root is **teased** from the socket. If the root is loose, but will not elevate, the second elevator can be placed on the opposite side of the root, and the root lifted from the socket. If the root tip is still attached by its periodontal ligament fibers, then you should use an elevator (#301), not Apex elevators, because the tips of the Apex elevators are not designed to be a displacement instrument. Apex elevator tips will bend or break if used to detach root tips.

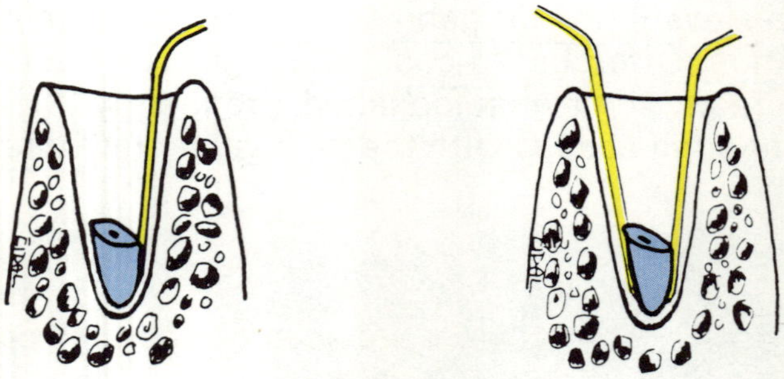

Figure II-14. Use of Apex elevators to tease root tip from socket.

Clinical Situation	Elevator(s)	Action
Removal of sectioned roots following sectioning	#30 & 31 (Cryer)	Wheel & axle; fulcrum placed on adjacent bone and is used with or without a purchase point
Removal of tooth or portion of tooth	#41 (Crane pick) (MOST DANGEROUS)	Wheel & axle; fulcrum placed on buccal bone, used with purchase point
Removal of maxillary third molars, both erupted and impacted	#73 & 74 Miller Potts	Wheel & axle and displacement; fulcrum placed on interseptal bone
Removal of larger single roots when forceps aren't preferred	#34-S & #46 (MOST COMMON)	Displacement
Luxating teeth prior to forceps application	#34-S & #46 #301 sometimes	Lever action; fulcrum placed on interseptal bone
Removal of medium size roots or medium size root tips when #34-S or #46 elevators are too large	#301, 302 & 303	Displacement
Removal of small root tips when tips have unobstructed pathway and are loose	Apex elevators (Root picks) (DELICATE)	Displacement

Figure II-15. Summary of use of elevators in oral surgery.

STUDY EXERCISES

The # ___ 30 ___ and ___ 31 ___ or Cryer elevators use the ___ WHEEL ___ and ___ AXLE ___ functional movements. They are used with or without the use of a ___ PURCHASE ___ point. They are used primarily for removing ___ ROOTS ___ when there is an adjacent empty ___ SOCKET ___. These elevators should be ___ SHARPENED ___ after each use.

The # ___ 41 ___ or Crane pick elevator can be extremely ___ DAMAGING ___ if used with uncontrolled forces. This elevator is used with a ___ WHEEL ___ and ___ AXLE ___ action with a fulcrum usually placed on ___ BUCCAL ___ bone. This elevator is usually used after the placement of a ___ PURCHASE POINT ___ ______ in the tooth or root.

The # ___ 73 ___ and ___ 74 ___ or Miller elevators and the ___ POTTS ___ elevators are used for the surgical removal of impacted maxillary ___ THIRD ___ molars.

The # ___ 34-S ___ and ___ 46 ___ are large shoehorn, straight elevators. These elevators are the most ___ COMMONLY ___ used elevators. Their main use is for the removal of ___ SINGLE ROOTS ___ ______ by their ___ DISPLACEMENT ___ effect. The main difference between these is that the # ___ 34-S ___ has a wider beak than the # ___ 46 ___.

The # 301, 302, and 303 elevators are used similarly to the #34-S and 46. These elevators are **NOT** used as WHEEL and AXLE or as a lever to pry teeth or roots. They are used by DISPLACEMENT action.

The APEX ELEVATORS or root picks have either a straight or angled SHANK. They are available in sets of different SIZES. Very small apex elevators are DELICATE instruments for the removal of SMALL DETACHED tips and should be used to tease out root tips rather than pry them out.

Complete the following summary chart by naming the elevator(s) to be used for each of the following clinical situations:

Clinical Situation	Elevator(s)	Action	Purchase Point Yes	Purchase Point No
Removal of sectioned roots following sectioning	30, 31 (CRYER)	WHEEL + AXLE	☑ or	☑
Removal of tooth or portion of tooth	41 (CRANE PICK)	WHEEL + AXLE	☑	☐
Removal of maxillary third molars, both erupted and impacted	73, 74 (MILLER) POTTS	WHEEL + AXLE; DISPLACEMENT	☐	☑
Removal of larger single roots when forceps aren't preferred	34-S, 46 (LARGE SHOEHORN, STRAIGHT ELEVATORS)	DISPLACEMENT	☐	☑
Luxating teeth prior to forceps application	34-S, 46, 301	LEVER ACTION	☐	☑
Removal of medium size roots or medium size root tips when #34-S or #46 elevators are too large	301, 302, 303	DISPLACEMENT	☐	☑
Removal of small root tips when tips have unobstructed pathway and are loose	APEX ELEVATORS (ROOT PICKS)	DISPLACEMENT	☐	☑

For Answers, see Figure II-15.

Unit III

MISCELLANEOUS SURGICAL INSTRUMENTS

Rongeurs
Chisels
Mallet
Curettes
Bone File
Periosteal Elevator
Scissors
Needle Holder
Suture Needles
Surgical Knife and Blades
Tissue Forceps
Transfer Forceps
Mouth Prop
Mosquito Hemostat
Retractor
Suction Tips
Surgical Burs
Rotary Cutting Instruments

PRETEST

- *Answer each question by circling the correct answer.*
- *If all questions are answered correctly, you have completed this unit and chapter.*
- *If you do not answer all questions correctly, read and study the content of this unit.*
- *The numbers in parentheses at the end of each question refer to the specific objective number from which this question was derived.*

Questions

Give the name of the instrument used in the following situations:

_______ 1. *To remove large amounts of bone as in alveoplasty procedures (01-03-01):*

a. *#12 bone file*
b. *#4A rongeurs*
c. *#5 rongeurs*
d. *#52 monobevel chisel*
e. *Molt or Lucas curettes*

_______ 2. *Which instrument is used with either the #2 bibevel chisel or sometimes with the #52 monobevel chisel (01-03-02)*

a. *#12 bone file*
b. *Surgical mallet*
c. *Dean scissors*
d. *Bard-Parker knife*
e. *None of the above*

_______ 3. *Which instrument is commonly used for removal of bone during a surgical extraction of teeth. Often they are so sharp that they can remove bone with hand pressure only (01-03-03).*

a. *#2 bibevel chisel*
b. *#52 monobevel chisel*
c. *#5 rongeurs*
d. *#34-S elevator*
e. *Both a & b*

_______ 4. *Which instrument is commonly used for removal of granulation tissue or enucleation of small cysts (01-03-04):*

a. *Periosteal elevator*
b. *Adson tissue forceps*
c. *6″ Kelly scissors*
d. *Molt or Lucas curettes*
e. *None of the above*

CURETTES

_______ 5. Which instrument is commonly used to smooth bone and remove bony spicules (01-03-05):
a. #4A rongeurs
b. #12 bone file
c. #5 rongeurs
d. Molt or Lucas curettes
e. None of the above

_______ 6. Which instrument is used to elevate periosteum from bone (01-03-06)
a. Lucas curettes
b. #9 Molt periosteal elevator
c. Hopkins periosteal elevator
d. Quinn periosteal elevator
e. Both b & c

_______ 7. Which instrument is used to trim tissue margins and for the removal of sutures (01-03-07)
a. Lucas curettes
b. Bard-Parker knife with #11 blade
c. Dean scissors
d. 6" Kelly scissors
e. Both c & d

_______ 8. Which instrument should be used to grasp suture needles (01-03-08):
a. 6" needle holder
b. Mosquito hemostats
c. Adson tissue forceps
d. Regular hemostats
e. None of the above

_______ 9. Which instrument is used to make incisions in mucoperiosteum (01-03-10):
a. #9 Molt periosteal elevator
b. Molt curette
c. Bard-Parker knife with #10 blade
d. Bard-Parker knife with #11, 12 or 15 blade
e. None of the above

_______ 10. Which instrument is used to support and stabilize soft tissue flaps during suturing (01-03-12)
a. Transfer forceps
b. Adson tissue forceps
c. Mosquito hemostat
d. Both b & c are correct
e. None of the above

_______ 11. Transfer forceps (01-03-13)
a. are used to transfer sterile items from supply area to surgical tray
b. are instruments enabling a "non-sterile" assistant to supply sterile items to surgical tray
c. should be sterilized daily
d. All of the above (a, b & c)
e. None of the above

_______ 12. An item used to support the mandible in an open position during posterior extraction procedures is (01-03-14):
a. A bite block
b. A mouth prop
c. A cotton roll
d. A folded gauze pad
e. None of the above

_______ 13. A many-purpose instrument used to clamp off blood vessels, aid in debridement, remove blades from surgical knives, and remove small root tips or bone fragments is (01-03-15):
a. Adson tissue forceps
b. Surgical clamp
c. Cotton pliers
d. Mosquito hemostat
e. None of the above

_______ 14. An instrument used to hold tissue flaps and cheeks out of the way during surgery is (01-03-16)

a. #9 periosteal elevator
b. Minnesota retractor
c. Austin retractor
d. Both b & c are correct
e. None of the above

_______ 15. Suction tips used for oral surgery differ from those used for general dentistry in that (01-03-18):

a. The orifice is larger
b. The orifice is smaller
c. They are longer and thinner
d. They deliver more suction
e. They are not different

_______ 16. A rotary cutting instrument should possess which of the following general characteristics (01-03-19):

a. Can be completely sterilized
b. Have high speed & torque
c. No air or oil exhaust into the wound
d. Possess a self-irrigating feature
e. All of the above

_______ 17. Which type of rotary cutting instrument is the most practical for use in a general dental office (01-03-21):

a. Turbo-jet
b. Stryker
c. Hall
d. Autoclavable high speed handpiece
e. None of the above

For each of the clinical situations described below, select a bur or burs that could be used from the following choices:

A. $33\frac{1}{2}$ inverted cone
B. Surgical acrylic or stump bur
C. #558 or #560 surgical length
D. #4 round bur surgical length
E. #170 surgical length
F. Tapered coarse diamond

_______ 18. Sectioning a maxillary first molar (01-03-23):

a. F
b. D
c. B
d. C, E #558 or 560 surgical length #170 surgical length.
e. C, E, F

_______ 19. Placement of purchase point (01-03-23):

a. B
b. D
d. F
e. E, D, C #170 surgical length #4 round bur surgical length #558 or 560 surgical length

_______ 20. Removal of a large exostosis (01-03-23):

a. E
b. A
c. B surgical acrylic or stump bur.
d. C
e. F

Answers

1. c	6. b	11. d	16. e
2. b	7. e	12. b	17. d
3. b	8. a	13. d	18. d
4. e	9. d	14. d	19. e
5. b	10. b	15. b	20. c

Unit III

MISCELLANEOUS SURGICAL INSTRUMENTS

In this unit we will discuss several miscellaneous instruments commonly used during minor oral surgery procedures. These instruments include:

Rongeurs	Scissors	Mosquito Hemostat
Chisels	Needle Holder	Retractor
Mallet	Surgical Knife & Blades	Suction Tips
Curettes	Tissue Forceps	Surgical Burs
Bone File	Transfer Forceps	Rotary Instruments
Periosteal Elevator	Mouth Prop	

RONGEURS

Although there are a number of rongeurs available, two commonly used are the #5 and #4A end-cutting rongeurs.

☐ #5 Rongeurs

The #5 rongeurs is a large-bladed, side-cutting rongeurs. It is often referred to as a bone forceps, since it cuts rather than pinches bone. This instrument provides a cleaner cut, and cuts over a greater surface. However, it requires significantly greater access than the #4A, and it poses a hazard, in that it has rather long blades which can very easily pinch and even cut lips and cheek tissue. This instrument is used primarily for major alveolar contouring (alveoplasty) when there is good access.

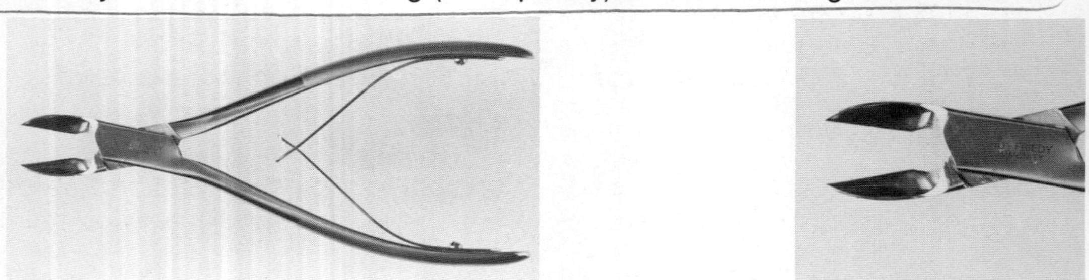

Figure III-1. A #5 Rongeurs.

☐ #4A Rongeurs and Blumenthal Rongeurs

The #4A rongeurs and Blumenthal rongeurs are both a side-cutting and end-cutting rongeurs. Either of these is usually the only rongeurs used by a general dentist. They cut bone by means of pinching. They are used primarily during minor alveoplasty since they require less access than the #5 rongeurs.

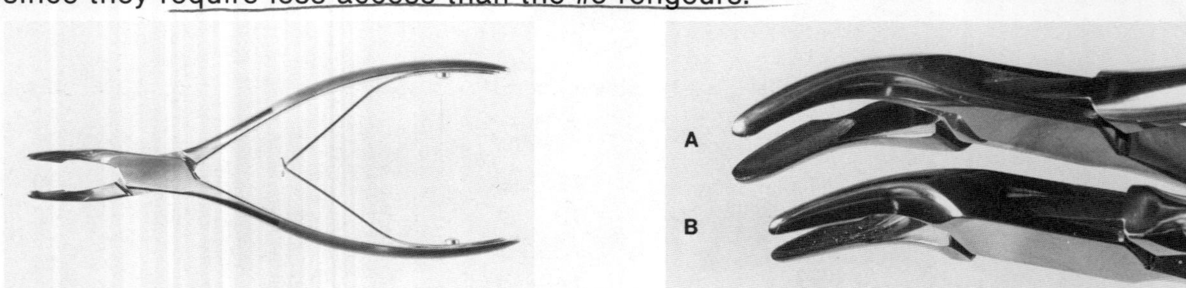

Figure III-2. A #4A Rongeurs. The close-up photo shows these two rongeurs to be virtually interchangeable. A. #4A. B. Blumenthal.

STUDY EXERCISES — Rongeurs

The two most commonly used rongeurs are the side-cutting or # 5 ______ *and the end-cutting or #* 4A ______ .

The #5, or SIDE – ______ *cutting rongeurs, is often referred to as a* BONE ______ *forceps since it* CUTS ______ *rather than* PINCHES ______ *bone. The #5 rongeurs requires (~~less~~/greater)* ______ *access and its long blades may* PINCH ______ *or even* CUT ______ *the lips or* CHEEKS ______ *. It is used for classical* ALVEOPLASTY ______ *, where there is good access and much bone is to be removed.*

Often the only rongeurs used by a general dentist is the # 4A ______ *or* BLUMENTHAL *cutting. It cuts bone by* PINCHING ______ *and may require (~~more~~/less)* ______ *access than the #* 5 ______ *side-cutting rongeurs.*

State which rongeurs you would be prepared to use for the following surgery request:

1. *Multiple extraction of periodontally involved mandibular arch — #19 through 29 followed by alveoplasty to establish smooth ridges for denture fabrication.* #5 ______

2. *Removal of cariously involved #30 in which #29, #31, #32 were previously extracted and a Kennedy Class I RPD is to be fabricated later.* # 4A ______

MALLET

☐ **Mallet — Surgical (Mead)**

The mallet is used with both the monobeveled and bibeveled (Wakefield and Gardner) chisels to either split teeth or remove bone. It is often equipped with a nylon head to soften the blow.

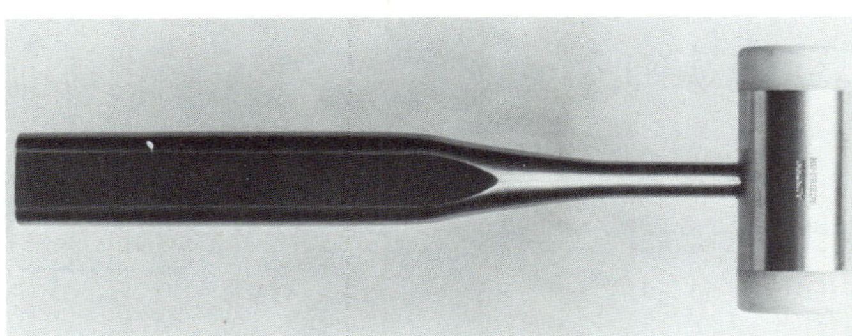

Figure III-3. A surgical mallet is used with a bibevel chisel and sometimes with a monobevel chisel.

A surgical mallet is used with a MONOBEVELED ______ *or* BIBEVELED (WAKEFIELD + GARDNER) ______ *chisel when* SPLITTING ______ *teeth or* REMOVAL OF ______ *bone.*

CHISELS

Chisels are used to either section teeth or to remove bone. To be effective, chisels must be kept sharp. You should sharpen chisels after each use. Chisels come in two forms as described below.

☐ **Bibevel #2 Chisel**

These are used to split teeth. It is ordinarily used in splitting mandibular third molars.

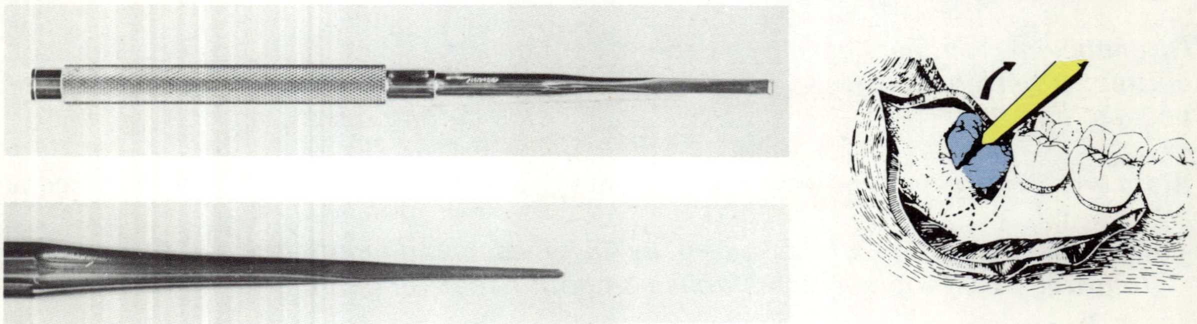

Figure III-4. A #2 bibevel chisel is used for splitting teeth.

☐ **Monobevel #52 Chisel**

This chisel is used for removing bone during impaction surgery and in the surgical extraction of teeth. Chisels of this type should be sharpened after each use. They should be so sharp that they can be used with hand pressure alone, if indicated.

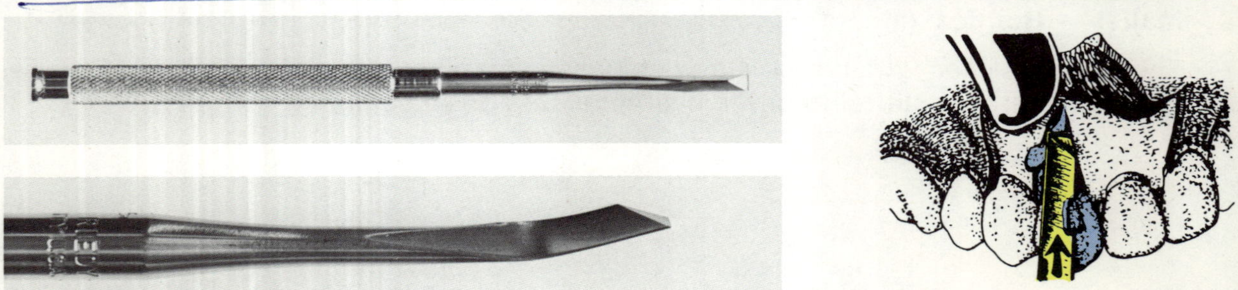

Figure III-5. A #52 monobevel chisel is used for bone removal.

Prior to elevation of a mesioangular impacted left third molar, the tooth is to be sectioned to remove the distal cusp. The chisel used for this would be #2 BI *-beveled.*

A lingual protuberance of bone is to be removed to eliminate an undercut area on the lingual cortical plate in the #18 area. Following the flap reflection, this bony protuberance may be removed with a #52 MONO *-bevel chisel. After each use, this chisel should be* SHARPENED *so as to cut bone with* HAND *pressure if needed.*

CURETTES

This instrument is primarily intended for curettage of granulomas and enucleation of small cysts. It is also used to debride sockets after extraction and to remove follicular tissue after the removal of impacted teeth. You will require a number of assorted sizes and shapes.

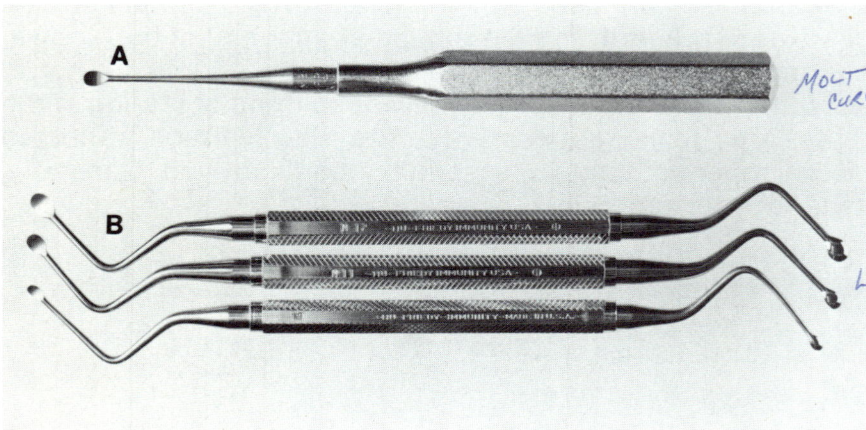

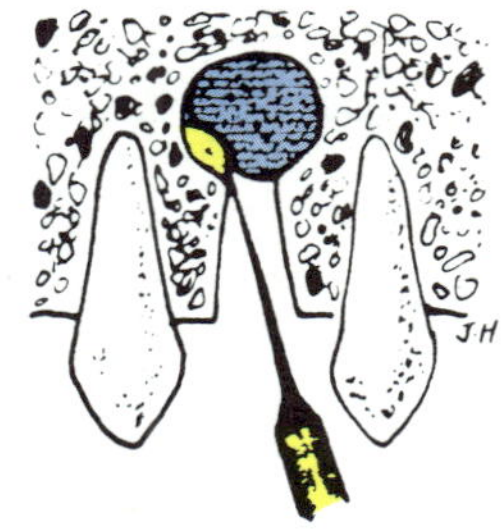

Notice that the back side of the curette is used to displace the cyst, and not to scrape the cyst from the bone.

Figure III-6. Curettes commonly used for oral surgery. A. Molt curette. B. Lucas curettes. Illustration shows use of a curette to remove a periapical cyst.

BONE FILE #12

This instrument is used for the final smoothing of bone. It should be emphasized that it is used only for the final smoothing, and not for gross bone reduction. Bone reduction should be achieved with the use of the rongeur forceps, and there should be very little need for the finishing touches with the bone file. The small end of the bone file is used most frequently and is used in a long sweeping stroke. The instrument cuts only on the pull stroke. It is important that this instrument be maintained in a sharp condition, otherwise it will only burnish the bone.

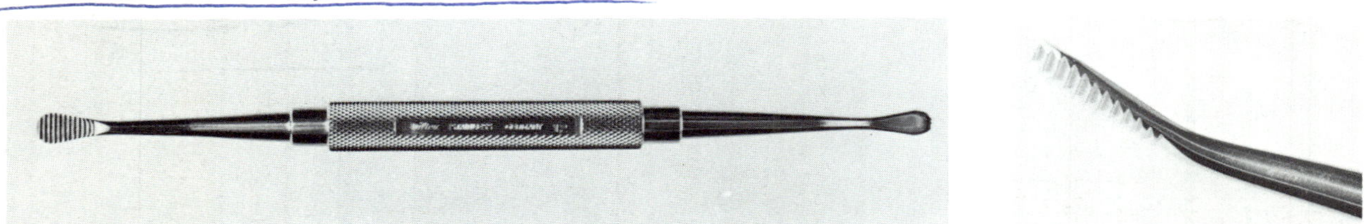

Figure III-7. A #12 bone file. Close-up photo shows that proper action of this file is obtained using a pull stroke.

Curettes are primarily intended for curettage of ____________ and enucleation of small ____________. Sockets also may be ____________ following extractions, except in the (maxillary/mandibular) ____________ molar area where the ____________ may possibly be involved.

A #____ file is for final ____________ of bone following ____________ reduction of bone by a ____________. This file files on the ____________ stroke and must be ____________ or else will ____________ the bone rather than file it.

PERIOSTEAL ELEVATOR

- ☐ **#9 (Molt)**
- ☐ **Hopkins**

These instruments are used primarily to reflect mucoperiosteum, and are occasionally used as retractors. They are used either with a push, pull, or pry stroke. The push and pry strokes are used primarily in severing the attachment of the gingiva, and the pull stroke is ordinarily used to reflect the more loosely attached gingiva. Great care should be used with these instruments to prevent splitting or tearing of the flap. If these instruments are not used carefully, the flap will be reflected supraperiosteally and the mucoperiosteum will essentially be destroyed. Generally, you will need only one type for your practice.

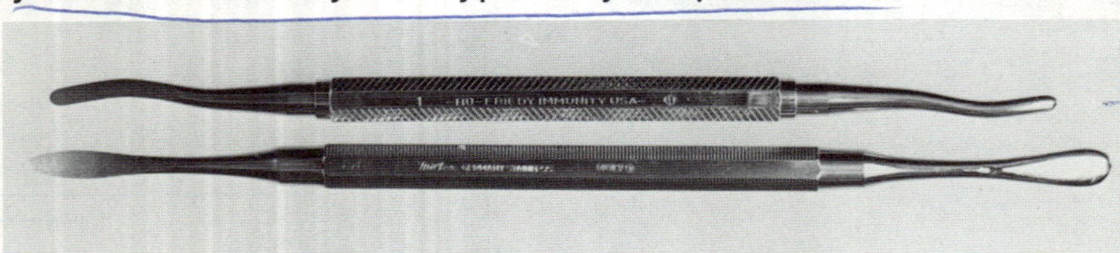

Hopkins

#9 (Molt)

Figure III-8. Periosteal elevators commonly used in oral surgery.

A # 9 (Molt) or a Hopkins elevator is used to reflect mucoperiosteum and may also be used as a retractor. push, pull and pry strokes are used; push and pry strokes are used primarily for severing the attachment of gingiva, pull stroke for reflecting loosely attached gingiva.

SCISSORS

Surgical scissors are used for trimming tissue or cutting sutures. Two scissors are commonly used; however, you will only need one type for your practice.

- ☐ **Kelly 6″ Curved Gum Scissors**

This instrument is intended as a universal-type scissors which can be used for trimming of wound margins and cutting of sutures. These scissors are slightly curved near the points. Left-handed models are also available.

- ☐ **Dean**

This scissors has a long curved handle that will lay flat along the alveolar ridge and offset straight blades.

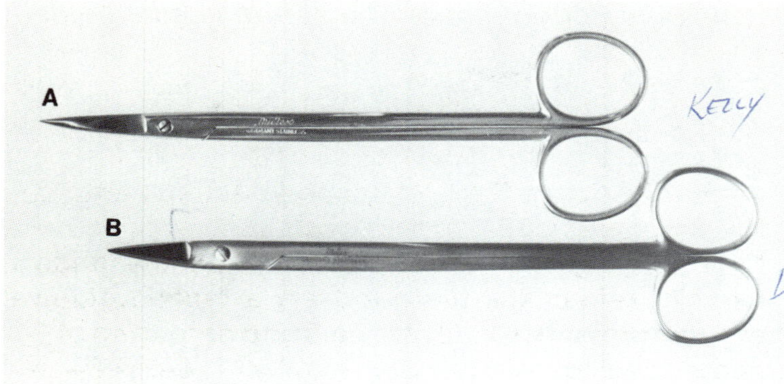

Figure III-9. Scissors commonly used for intraoral surgery. A. Kelly. B. Dean.

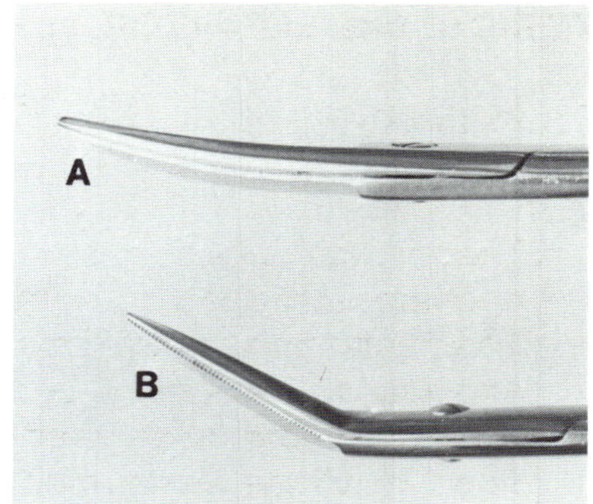

Figure III-10. Close-up view. A. Kelly. B. Dean.

Scissors are used for ____TRIMMING____ *tissue or cutting of* ____SUTURES____ *.*
Two commonly used surgical scissors are the ____KELLY____ *and the* ____DEAN____ *.*

NEEDLE HOLDER

A 6-inch suture needle holder is recommended when suturing intraoral incisions. The preferred method of holding the needle holder is to place your thumb and ring or third finger through the holes, and then to place your index finger along the shaft. This may feel awkward at first (you may be tempted not to place your fingers through the holes, or to place your index finger through the other hole), but it is necessary to hold the needle holder correctly in order to open and close the instrument while suturing. The art of suturing is perhaps the last to be mastered during surgery. One of the reasons is failure to master the correct grasp of the needle holder.

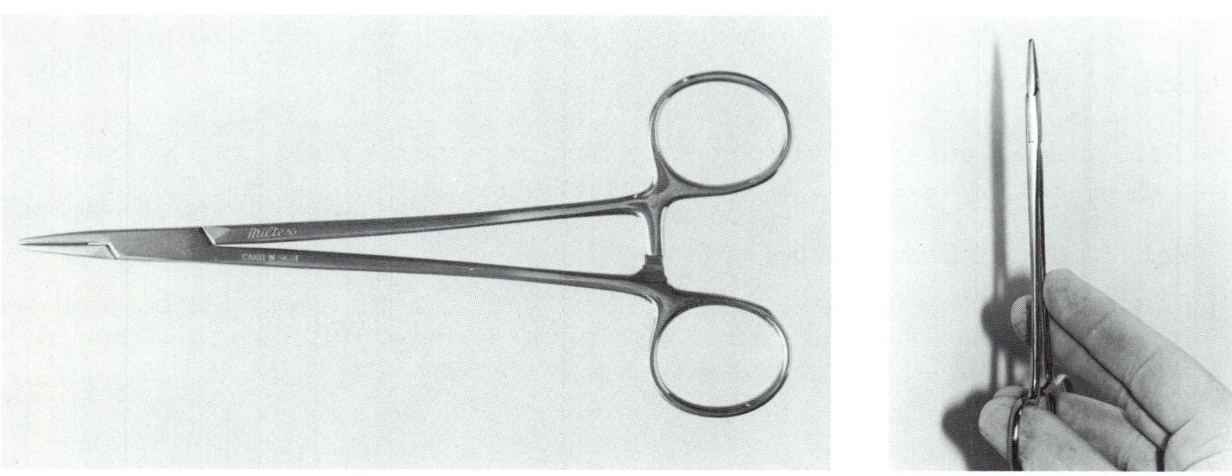

Figure III-11. A 6″ needle holder and correct grasp of this instrument.

Which of the following illustrations shows the correct grasp of a suture needle holder?

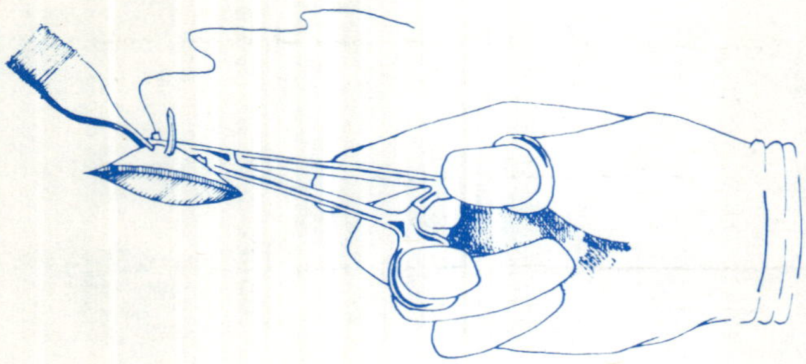

A

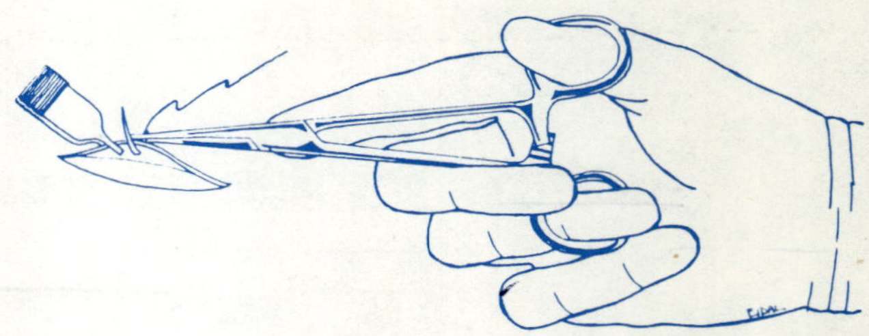

B

Briefly describe the placement of your thumb, index finger, middle finger, ring finger and little finger when correctly using a needle holder.

Thumb: PLACED THRU HANDLE-HOLE

Index finger: ALONG THE SHAFT

Middle finger: BENT BACK

Ring finger: PLACED THRU HANDLE-HOLE

Little finger: BENT BACK

Why is the above placement advantageous? NECESSARY TO HOLD THE NEEDLE HOLDER CORRECTLY AND TO OPEN + CLOSE THE INSTRUMENT WHILE SUTURING.

See Figure III-11 for correct answer.

SURGICAL KNIFE & BLADES

#3 Bard-Parker Knife Handle with Blades #11, #12, and #15

The #15 blade is the standard blade used for almost all oral surgical procedures. The #11 blade is pointed and is used for incision and drainage procedures. The #12 blade is "hooked" and can reach some otherwise inaccessible regions such as the tuberosity region. The #12b blade incises on both sides. The #10 blade is not used for intraoral surgery.

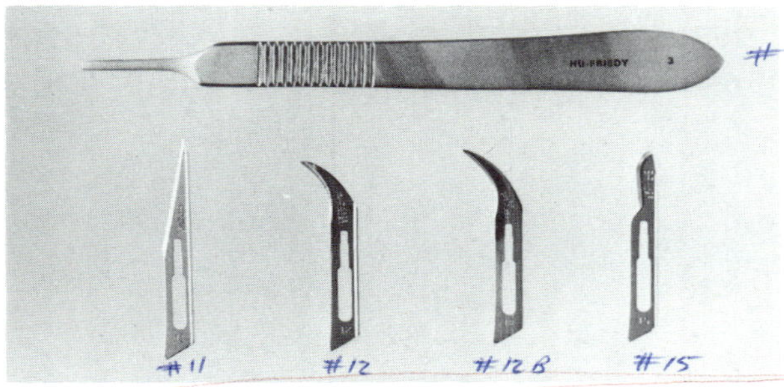

Figure III-12. #3 Bard-Parker knife handle and #11, 12, 12b and 15 blades commonly used for intraoral surgery.

Care should be taken when changing blades so that you (or your assistant) do not injure yourself. Place the blade onto the knife handle using a needle holder. When removing the blade, grasp the lower end with a needle holder, lift this edge, and slide the blade off the handle.

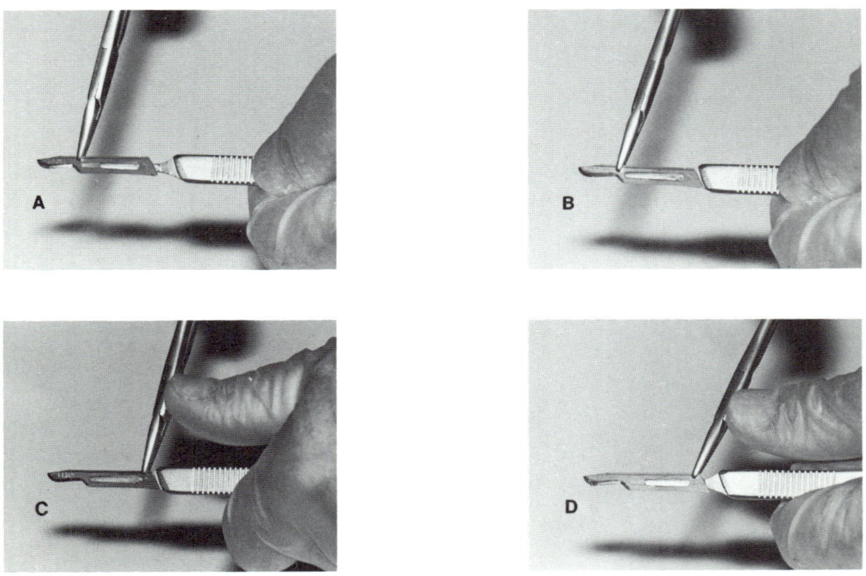

Figure III-13. **Steps for placement and removal of surgical blades from knife handle. A. Grasp middle of blade with needle holder. B. Slide blade onto latch mechanism on handle. C. Clamp blade flange near end of blade with needle holder and disengage lock. D. Slide blade off of handle.**

STUDY EXERCISES

Three blade styles used in oral surgery are the #15 *for almost all* oral surgical *procedures,* #11 *for* incision & drainage*, and the* #12 *for* poorly accessible *regions.*

Blades should be removed with a needle holder *and not with your fingers.*

TISSUE FORCEPS

There are a variety of tissue forceps used in oral surgery for supporting and stabilizing soft tissue flaps, usually during suturing. They are available with and without "teeth."

☐ Adson

The Adson tissue forceps with "teeth" are generally used in oral surgery to support flaps, enabling the suture needle to penetrate the flap at a 90° angle. They are also useful in supporting tissue in biopsy procedures. When used in biopsies, you should use extreme care to avoid crushing or otherwise destroying the tissue specimen.

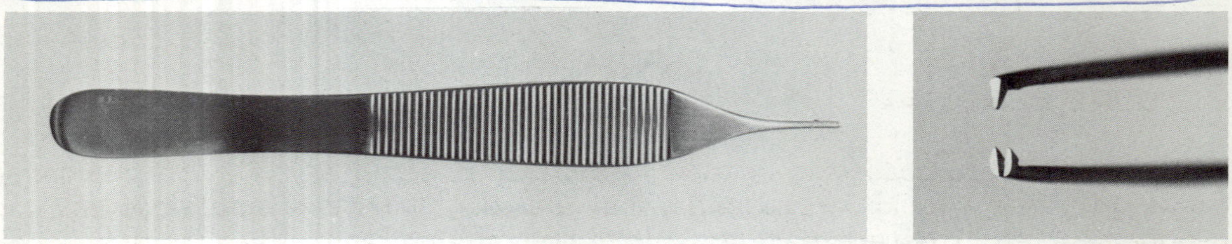

Figure III-14. Adson tissue forceps.

The main uses for tissue forceps during oral surgery are to SUPPORT *and* STABILIZE *soft tissue flaps, usually during* SUTURING*. During a biopsy procedure, tissue forceps can be useful in* SUPPORTING *the tissue. Great care should be taken so as not to* CRUSH *or otherwise* DESTROY *the tissue specimen.*

TRANSFER FORCEPS

This instrument enables a "non-sterile" member of the team to place sterile instruments and supplies on the surgical tray. The transfer forceps are usually kept in a special receptacle designed to hold a disinfecting solution. Since it is difficult not to contaminate disinfecting solution, it is best to keep the receptacles dry and autoclave the transfer forceps daily.

Figure III-15. Use of transfer forceps for aseptic transfer of materials during surgery.

Transfer forceps allow a NON-STERILE *-person to place* STERILE *instruments and supplies on the surgical tray. This instrument is usually kept in a special receptacle designed to contain a* DISINFECTING *solution. It is best (to fill/not fill)* ________ *the container with disinfectant. The recommended procedure is to* KEEP THE RECEPTACLES DRY AND AUTOCLAVE THE TRANSFER FORCEPS DAILY*. The reason for this is that* IT IS DIFFICULT NOT TO CONTAMINATE THE DISINFECTING SOLUTION*.*

MOUTH PROP

A mouth prop, such as the McKesson, is essential during extractions in the mandibular posterior sextant to minimize temporomandibular joint trauma and for patients who are sedated, since it is difficult for them to keep their mouth open over an extended period of time. Mouth props are available in several sizes. Mouth props can also be of help when treating over-anxious patients to assist you in minimizing operating time.

Mouth props are essential for extractions in the MAND. POSTERIOR ______ *sextant and especially for patients who are* SEDATED. ______.

MOSQUITO HEMOSTAT

These are multi-purpose instruments. In general surgery, they are used primarily to clamp off blood vessels. In exodontia, they are used to remove small root tips, aid in debridement, etc. They are manufactured in both straight and curved models.

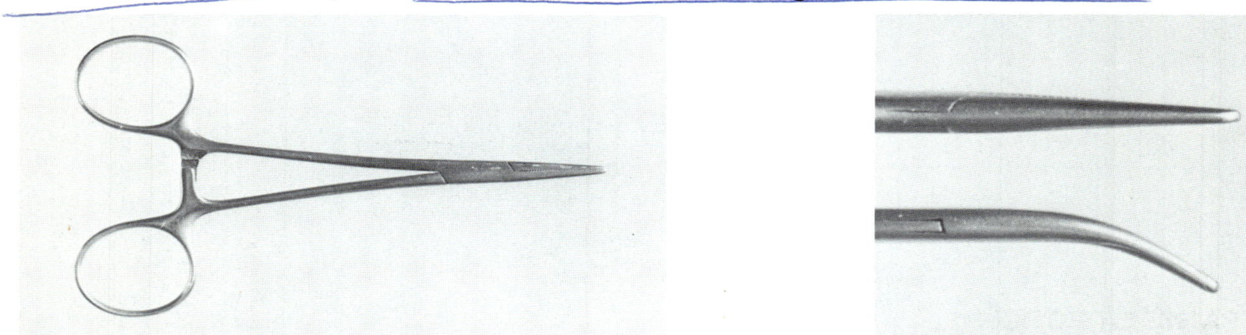

Figure III-16. Mosquito hemostat. Close up shows both straight and curved beaks.

RETRACTORS

Retractors are used to hold mucoperiosteal flaps, cheeks, lips and tongue away from the surgical area. This improves visibility and protects these tissues from injury.

- ☐ **Minnesota Retractor**
- ☐ **Austin Retractor**

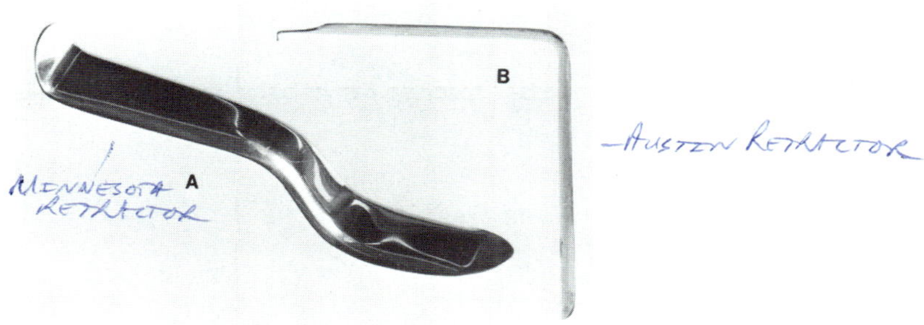

Figure III-17. Tissue retractors used for intraoral surgery. A. Minnesota retractor. B. Austin retractor.

Two commonly used retractors are the ____________________ and ____________________. They are used to retract ____________________ and ____________________ while you are performing surgery.

SUCTION TIPS

Suction tips used for oral surgery differ from those used in general dentistry. They are designed to provide efficient suction in small areas without grabbing your surgical flaps. The orifice is generally smaller than suction tips used for general dentistry. The handle and tubing entering your surgical field should be of a sterilizable material.

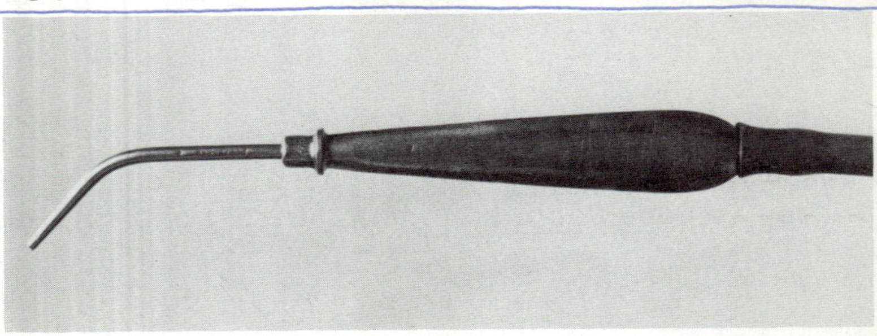

Figure III-18. Surgical aspirator.

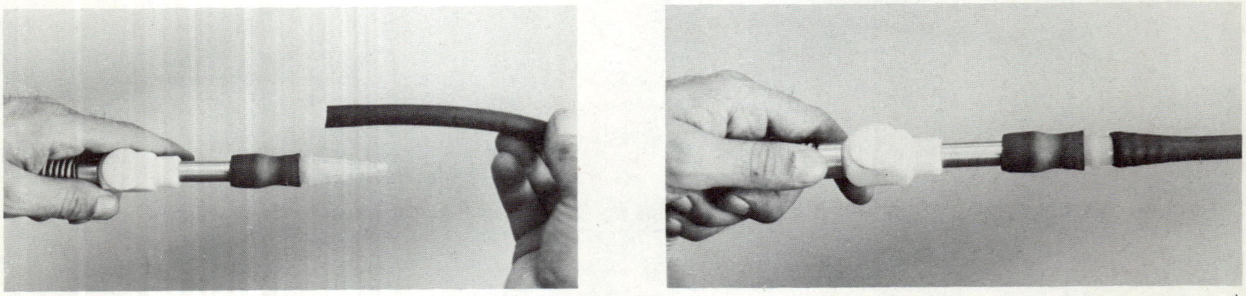

Figure III-19. Adaptation of a typical aspirator handle used in general dentistry to obtain a sterile surgical field.

SURGICAL BURS

Burs are used frequently during oral surgical procedures for a variety of applications as summarized below. **Surgical length burs** have a longer shank than burs used in restorative dentistry and are especially useful when sectioning teeth through furcations because the longer shank enables you to keep your handpiece out of your visual field. A great variety of burs are available to fit the chuck mechanisms of rotary cutting instruments. **Carbide burs** will remain sharper for a longer period of time than steel burs. **Diamond stones** are rarely used for oral surgery because they are less efficient for tooth sectioning and are more expensive.

Bur Type	Bur Numbers	Uses
Straight fissure burs	#558-560	These burs are used to remove bone, section teeth, or to place purchase points. Use of an end-cutting fissure bur will meet all of your needs when removing teeth.
Tapered fissure burs	#702, 703, 704	
End-cutting fissure burs	#1158, 1171	
Round burs	#4	Placement of purchase point
Acrylic or stump burs		Removal of exostosis or torus.

Figure III-20. Burs commonly used for intraoral surgery.

ROTARY CUTTING INSTRUMENTS

An acceptable rotary cutting instrument is an indispensable item for performing surgical procedures. It is used for sectioning teeth, removal of root tips, removal of bone around and over impacted teeth.

In making recommendations for equipment which ultimately can be used for general practice, we are faced with a real dilemma, since there is no ideal equipment available which is 100% practical for the general practitioner to purchase.

First, let us consider the features that the ideal rotary cutting equipment would possess:

- Can be completely sterilized by acceptable methods
- High speed
- High torque
- No air or oil exhaust into the wound
- Possess a self-irrigating attachment
- Reasonable size — not too bulky
- Adaptable to equipment used in general practice

Several systems have been designed for use in facilities primarily emphasizing oral surgery such as hospital clinics and oral surgery specialty practices. These systems are expensive, but worth the investment if heavily used. The following is a brief description of three of these systems.

- **Turbo-Jet**

  The turbo-jet is a self-contained water powered system which provides about 100,000 rpm and high torque to the surgical bur. The handpiece is completely autoclavable; however, the tubing is not. Care should be exercised when using a turbo-jet to avoid abrasion of lips. The water supply for both turning the rotor and irrigating the surgical site is held in a reservoir in the unit. Water should be changed daily to avoid growth of microorganisms. This also could be a drawback if this item is not used frequently.

- **Hall Air Turbine**

  This also is completely autoclavable. From the point of view of complete aseptic technique, this instrument offers some advantages since the tubing, as well as the handpiece, is autoclavable. It uses a special air source, either a 120 psi line or a nitrogen cylinder. The overall cost, as well as the special provision for high pressure air, make this unit impractical for most office uses in general dentistry.

- **Stryker Drill**

  The Stryker is very similar to the Hall air turbine. It is primarily intended for use in the operating room. Like the Hall drill, it is an excellent system, but its cost will most likely deter most general practitioners.

Air Rotors Used for General Dentistry

Generally speaking, high speed and low speed dental handpieces are not ideally suited for oral surgery.

- **High Speed Air Rotors**

  While many high speed handpieces are now autoclavable, they exhaust air into surgical wounds and can cause air embolisms to form in soft tissue. Another drawback is that they use water supplied from the dental unit. This water can be highly contaminated and water spray should not be used (see **Chapter 5, Asepsis in Oral Surgery).** The chuck mechanism for changing burs should also be sterilizable.

  One high speed handpiece, the "Impact-Air 45," manufactured by Innovators, Inc., is gaining in popularity among oral surgeons and general practitioners. It fulfills most of the criteria listed above for an ideal handpiece. It is autoclavable and fits all standard air lines. It does not exhaust into the wound and can be modified to use sterile water or saline for irrigation. This handpiece is constructed with an off-set head, allowing greater access to posterior areas.

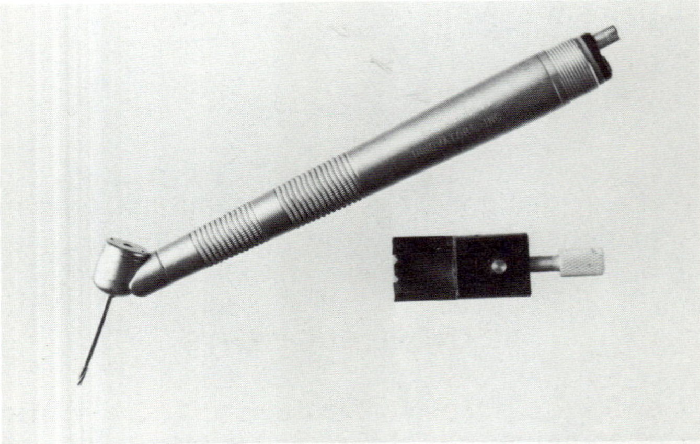

Figure III-20. Impact-Air 45 high speed handpiece is an example of an acceptable air rotor for use during oral surgery procedures in a general dental office.

  This handpiece is reasonably priced and well suited for use in a general dental office. For the occasional exodontist this handpiece can easily be preserved in a sterile wrap and used when needed.

  Several other manufacturers have produced autoclavable high speed air rotors which can be used; however, models designed for restorative dentistry generally have lower torque and are thus less efficient for tooth sectioning during surgical procedures. They may, however, be easier to use in areas of the mouth anterior to the third molar region. You should avoid use of fiber optic handpieces at this time because they currently cannot be sterilized.

- **Slow Speed Air Rotors**

  Some slow speed handpieces are also autoclavable and acceptable for surgery; however, they are somewhat slow for efficient use.

STUDY EXERCISES

The ideal features for a rotary cutting instrument are:

1. CAN BE COMPLETELY STERILIZED BY ACCEPTABLE METHODS
2. HIGH SPEED
3. HIGH TORQUE
4. (NO) AIR OR OIL EXHAUST INTO THE WOUND
5. REASONABLE SIZE
6. ADAPTABLE TO EQUIPMENT USED IN GENERAL DENTISTRY

Three air rotor systems frequently found in oral surgery clinics include:

1. TURBO-JET
2. HALL AIR TURBINE
3. STRYKER DRILL

The major drawback for these systems is THEY ARE EXPENSIVE.

Most high speed and low speed dental handpieces (~~are~~/are (not)) viewed by oral surgeons to be acceptable for oral surgery. The major drawbacks for these handpieces include:

1. EXHAUST AIR INTO SURGICAL WOUNDS → CAUSE AIR EMBOLI
2. USE WATER SUPPLIED BY THE DENTAL UNIT → CAN BE CONTAMINATED
3. CHUCK MECHANISM IS NOT STERILIZABLE
4. SLOW SPEED HANDPIECES ARE TOO SLOW FOR EFFICIENT USE.

ACKNOWLEDGMENTS

We wish to extend a special thanks to: **Dr. James H. Quinn,** Department of Oral & Maxillofacial Surgery, Louisiana State University School of Dentistry for his enthusiasm and technical assistance and to the **Hu-Friedy Instrument Manufacturers,** 3118 N. Rockwell St., Chicago, Illinois 60618, and **Miltex Instrument Company,** 6 Ohio Drive, Lake Success, New York 11092, who both graciously supplied instruments for our photographs in this chapter.

NOTES